HEALTH
GAP

The

HEALTH GAP

Beyond Pregnancy and Reproduction

Jennifer Kitts
and
Janet Hatcher Roberts

INTERNATIONAL DEVELOPMENT RESEARCH CENTRE
Ottawa • Cairo • Dakar • Johannesburg • Montevideo • Nairobi • New Delhi • Singapore

Published by the International Development Research Centre
PO Box 8500, Ottawa, ON, Canada K1G 3H9

© International Development Research Centre 1996

Canadian Cataloguing in Publication Data

Kitts, Jennifer

The health gap : beyond pregnancy and reproduction

"There is clearly a need for further interdisciplinary research on various aspects of
women's health to integrate a gender perspective into the research protocol as it is
conceived, carried out, analyzed, and disseminated." — Preface
Includes bibliographical references.

ISBN: 0-88936-772-8

1. Women — Health and hygiene — Developing countries — Congresses.
I. Hatcher Roberts, Janet.
II. International Development Research Centre (Canada).
III. Title.

RA778.A2K57 1996   613'.04244'097124   C96-980022-3

A microfiche edition is available.

Contents

Preface

Between October 1993 and January 1995, the International Development Research Centre (IDRC) sponsored a series of four regional workshops on gender, health, and sustainable development. The workshops were held in Nairobi, Kenya (5–8 October 1993), Montevideo, Uruguay (26–29 April 1994), Bridgetown, Barbados (6–9 December 1994), and Singapore (23–26 January 1995). These workshops evolved from the growing understanding that women in developing countries face significantly different health risks than men and also experience different constraints when resolving their health problems. They also stemmed from the recognition that major gaps exist in our understanding of gender and health, largely because much previous research, to some extent, bypassed women.

The workshops brought together scientists and social scientists with expertise in a wide range of areas of women's health. Participants came from Bangladesh, Barbados, Bolivia, Brazil, Cambodia, Cameroon, Chile, China, Colombia, Commonwealth of Dominica, Costa Rica, Dominican Republic, Ecuador, Ethiopia, Ghana, Guyana, India, Indonesia, Japan, Jamaica, Kenya, Korea, Laos, Malaysia, Mexico, Mongolia, Myanmar (formerly Burma), Nicaragua, Nigeria, Paraguay, Peru, the Philippines, Singapore, South Africa, St Lucia, Tanzania, Thailand, Trinidad, Uganda, Uruguay, Venezuela, Viet Nam, Zambia, and Zimbabwe. Representatives from a number of different international agencies were present, including staff from IDRC.

The workshops were designed to examine four priority areas that urgently require more research from a gender perspective: AIDS (acquired immune deficiency syndrome), health and the working environment, tropical diseases, and barriers to quality health care. Additional issues were integrated into each workshop based on regional priorities — nutrition was given special attention at the Caribbean workshop, health issues of indigenous peoples were explored at the Latin American workshop, and the effects of war on women's health were addressed in Asia. The participants also sought to translate their insights into recommendations for future research to promote health and welfare for all. Specific workshop objectives were:

+ To encourage health researchers, nongovernmental organizations (NGOs), and policymakers to incorporate within their research, activities, and policy work, the interrelated dimensions of gender and sustainable development;

- ✦ To share gender and health research from various parts of the developing world;
- ✦ To examine methodologies for gender and health research;
- ✦ To identify key gaps in gender and health research;
- ✦ To discuss health within the broad context of the conditions and forces that influence the lives of women and men; and
- ✦ To compare and contrast the issues facing various countries in the developing world and the strategies used to overcome obstacles to health.

The exchange of insights and experiences among participants at each regional workshop was highly constructive and beneficial. The cross-fertilization of ideas and perspectives that resulted from bringing together participants with different areas of expertise from various parts of each region was particularly enriching.

Although each workshop was unique, common issues, concerns, and recommendations clearly emerged. This book synthesizes the presentations, discussions, and group work undertaken at the four workshops and pulls together the cumulative wisdom of the participants. Additional materials have also been consulted and integrated into the synthesis. In particular, information from papers submitted to essay competitions between 1991 and 1994 sponsored by IDRC and the World Health Organization (WHO) Special Programme for Research and Training in Tropical Diseases (TDR) on gender and tropical diseases was incorporated. Papers presented at a October 1994 workshop on the quality of health care for women in developing countries (sponsored by WHO and the Ford Foundation) were also reviewed.

There is clearly a need for further interdisciplinary research on various aspects of women's health to integrate a gender perspective into the research protocol as it is conceived, carried out, analyzed, and disseminated. Researchers and organizations from around the world can achieve significant advancements in research in this area by working cooperatively and consolidating their experiences and results. It is hoped that this publication will serve as a basis for further dialogue and initiatives aimed at improving the health and well-being of women and inspire more collaborative work and networking among biomedical and social science researchers.

Jennifer Kitts
Janet Hatcher Roberts
January 1996

Introduction

An Elusive Right

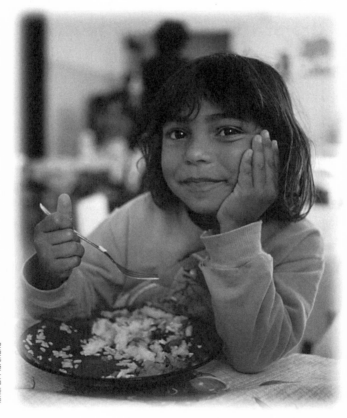

*Why should we look at women separate from men? One might
point to a few pertinent facts: women have special health
problems that men do not experience; women are more
vulnerable to certain conditions than are men; some health
conditions are less easily detected in women; women's health
directly affects child survival chances; and women's needs are
often neglected if not specifically identified.*

— Eva M. Rathgeber, International Development Research Centre,
Regional Office for Eastern and Southern Africa, Nairobi, Kenya

GENDER INEQUITIES IN HEALTH

Health, a basic human right that is vital to sustainable development, eludes
the majority of women. Although women in most societies live longer than
men (for biological reasons), women often suffer greater burdens of illness
and disability than their male counterparts. There are sharp inequities in
health in both developing and industrialized countries; however, the disparities are more pronounced in developing nations (World Bank 1993). For
example, about half a million women die every year from the complications
of pregnancy and childbirth. Most of these deaths are preventable with simple technologies that have been available for decades. Maternal mortality
ratios (maternal deaths per 100 000 live births) are, on average, 30 times
higher (and in some cases are 200 times higher) in developing countries than
in high-income countries (World Bank 1993).

As a result of visible and invisible discrimination, subordination, and
undervaluation experienced throughout life, women are more vulnerable to
poverty, poor nutrition, preventable diseases, uncontrolled fertility, premature death, violence, disability, alienation, and loneliness. The quality of
women's lives is further impaired by insufficient education, poor housing and
sanitation, long hours of work in physically demanding and often dangerous
conditions, inadequate and inaccessible health-care services, and lack of
family and community support.

As described by Seble Dawitt (1994):

> Harmful cultural practices perpetuated on women and girls ... include
> child marriage and early pregnancy, forced feeding before a wedding,
> nutritional taboos, particularly during pregnancy, certain birthing prac-
> tices, female genital mutilation, less food, education and health care for
> girls, dowry and bride price, widow inheritance, and female infanticide ....
> The result for individual women and girls is mitigation of their health or
> their quality of life. What all these practices have in common is that they
> evolve from, or are in reaction to, the preference for male children.

Gender inequities, and the preference for male children, sometimes starts even before birth. Diagnostic techniques, such as amniocentesis, chorionic villus sampling, and targeted ultrasound, have made it possible for parents to discover the sex of the fetus and to terminate the pregnancy if they had hoped for a child of the other sex. In a number of countries (such as China, India, and Korea), the selective abortion of female fetuses is becoming more and more common as a result of these new technologies (RCNRT 1993; Oh 1995).

GAPS IN GENDER AND HEALTH RESEARCH

In *The Female Client and the Health Care Provider*, H.V. Wyatt (1995) points out:

> Since 1945, there have been several hundred papers published on the topic of polio in India, covering immunization, prevalence of acute and residual paralysis, and rehabilitation. Yet no paper discusses differencing related to gender. Even data that might have been analyzed by gender are always presented as a total ... [researchers] carry out extensive house to house surveys to locate disabled children — and then file their results in such a way that differences related to gender cannot be examined.

Major gaps exist in our understanding of gender and health, largely because much research in the past has to some extent bypassed women (Rathgeber 1994a). In many countries, there is a serious lack of rigorous sex-disaggregated research. Health research has tended to overlook the specific consequences of disease and illness on women and men and neglected to examine fully the different social, cultural, and economic contexts within which women and men work and live (Rathgeber and Vlassoff 1993).

Studies have also largely failed to investigate the impact that the physical and biological differences between women and men have on the

[In Korea] many induced abortions are performed because the sex of the fetus is thought to be female. Recent medical technological advances now allow for the identification of fetal sex during the first trimester of pregnancy. As a result of the high number of abortions of female fetuses, there is now a severe imbalance of the sexes.

— Kasil Oh, Yonsei University, Seoul, Korea

> *[It is a mistake] to assume that the norm of male experience is equally applicable to women — that women have the same attitudes and perceptions, the same opportunities and lack of opportunities, and the same needs as their male counterparts.*
>
> — Eva M. Rathgeber, International Development Research Centre, Regional Office for Eastern and Southern Africa, Nairobi, Kenya

epidemiology and etiology of disease. Medical research tends to have a male bias (Rosser 1991), and health research (other than reproductive health) is often carried out on male subjects and the results are assumed to be relevant to both women and men. As an illustration, women have not been included in clinical trials of the extent to which azidothymidine (AZT) inhibits the progression of AIDS, and researchers therefore do not know how well AZT works on women. Women often respond differently to treatment, metabolize drugs differently, and, according to Donna Stewart of the University of Toronto, "are not just men with menstrual cycles" (Priest 1994, p. A1).

Despite the fact that women make up a rapidly increasing number of those infected with HIV (human immunodeficiency virus), women remain at a disadvantage regarding diagnosis, treatment, and care because of gender inequities in health research (Strebel 1994). Hankins and Handley (1992, p. 967) argued:

> A concerted effort on the part of clinicians, researchers, funding agencies, and decision-makers is required for redressing the inequities in both the gender-specific knowledge of the natural history, progression, and outcome of HIV disease and the adequacy of medical and psychosocial care for women with HIV infection. The unique features of HIV infection in women have been subject to both scientific neglect and policy void.

The gender dimensions of many other areas of health research beyond AIDS have also been neglected. In the area of tropical diseases, for example (Rathgeber and Vlassoff 1993, p. 513):

> Both biomedical and social research on the effects of tropical diseases on women has taken a narrow perspective. It has focused primarily on sex differences, particularly related to pregnancy and reproduction, and has not examined these in relation to broader social roles and responsibilities.

Timoteo and Llanos-Cuentas (1994) reported that, in a search for studies related to gender and tropical diseases in Peru, they discovered an overwhelming absence of literature on the subject. For example, in bibliographies on leishmaniasis, there were very few studies related to how this disease affects women and men differentially from a socioeconomic and cultural perspective. Even if sex was identified as a variable in studies, there was little or no analysis of the impact of broader gender relations.

The health implications of women's work is yet another area of study that has been highly neglected in research. The limited research has tended to focus on the reproductive health effects of work, rather than on the health of women themselves. Furthermore, there is a dearth of research that explores the direct health effects of women's heavy workloads in and around the household and in the informal work force.

> *Health services for women usually emphasize and cater to the reproductive health needs of women, and little effort is made by the health sector to help women realize that they are persons in their own right, with their own personal health needs. Women's health needs are given less attention within the structure of health-service provision than the health needs of children. Their quality is poorer, and more often than not, women's needs are subordinated to population-control programs.*
>
> — S.A. Udipi and M.A. Varghese, SNDT Women's University, Bombay, India

BEYOND PREGNANCY AND REPRODUCTIVE HEALTH

One of the goals of these workshops was to adopt a holistic approach to women's health and to place greater emphasis on the quality of well-being of women's lives outside the sphere of fertility and reproduction. In the past, when women's health has received attention, "reproductive health and women's health have been treated in general as if conterminous" (Manderson 1994, p. 2), and more concern has been placed on children resulting from pregnancy than on women themselves. The extent to which women's health and well-being affects perinatal and infant mortality, for example, has been a key focal point. In the area of AIDS research, most early studies in women were largely restricted to preventing transmission of HIV from an infected mother to her child (Cohen 1995), and women themselves were neglected from the beginning of the epidemic.

Commentators have noted that the focus on women when discussing contraception and family planning has had more to do with containing population growth than enhancing the health and well-being of women. Research in this domain has been motivated largely by widespread concerns about the need to curtail high birth rates and control population growth, "rather than by concern with women's health as a good in itself" (Vlassoff 1994, p. 1250).

In service delivery, as well, programs for women have been geared toward the reproductive role of women and a narrow family-planning focus. Women's medical services often have a lower priority within the structure of health-service provision than those for children and men, and their quality is poorer (Udipi and Varghese 1995). This perpetuates the notion that women's needs are secondary to others. Women are viewed "first as mothers or future mothers," whereas men's health "is never defined from a family or fathering perspective" (Rathgeber and Vlassoff 1993, p. 514).

The fields of both medicine and public health have perpetuated the classic androcentric view of woman that focuses on her reproductive capacity and circumscribes her to the singular role of mother.

— Jaime Breilh, Health Research Consultancy Centre, Quito, Ecuador

Richters (1994, p. 42) called for a deconstruction of "the ideology that women's sole natural destiny is to fulfil the biological role of procreation." Women must be seen as human beings with needs and desires that relate to them personally as women. Research with regard to women should aim to empower them as individuals, as people in their own right, without always looking at their role as nurturers.

Research should also cover the entire life span of women, "from the fetus threatened by malnutrition and gender selection to the post-menopausal woman debilitated and marginalized by osteoporosis."[1] Health research and policies must incorporate "the full range of [women's] needs and activities and all the discomforts and illnesses that they face" (Richters 1994, p. 43). As Denise Eldemire (1995), from the University of the West Indies, correctly points out:

> The older woman has been essentially ignored, menopausal issues not addressed, and the contribution of older women as grandmothers, child carers and rearers, and housekeepers not given adequate recognition. Such activities are a resource and a contribution to development because they allow other family members to be productive. They also serve to raise the next generation of workers.

---

[1] Comment of V. Wee at the IDRC workshop on gender, health, and sustainable development held in Singapore, 23–26 January 1995.

Chapter I

Gender, Health, and Development

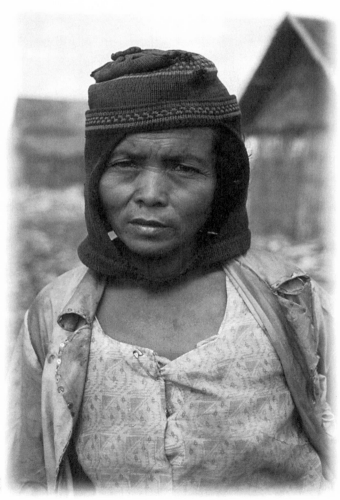

Health has to be a necessary input to, and goal of, development. It is necessary that women are healthy in order for them to participate fully in development as workers, mothers, and family and community members. Besides being recipients of health care, women are also providers and promoters of health.

— K. Soin, Member of Parliament, Republic of Singapore

GENDER

In most if not all societies, the socioeconomic relations between women and men are largely unequal and hierarchical. The disparity between women and men can be seen in the legitimization of a sexual division of labour beyond purely biological roles in the household and the formal work force and in the practices that are gender discriminatory in other societal institutions (Tsikata 1994). Women have fewer educational opportunities than men and receive unequal distribution of land and access to resources such as food and health care (Wee 1995).

The traditional theory explaining the emergence of separate roles for women and men posited that there were biologically determined differences between females and males. However, the belief that there are fundamental and immutable differences between women and men has been thoroughly challenged by feminist commentators. They have argued that sexuality is in fact socially constructed and historically located within a matrix of inter-secting social, economic, and cultural factors (Caplan 1987).

Gender relations are not biologically determined; rather, they are based on differential relations of power in which patriarchy exerts substantial control over women in a variety of spheres (Strebel 1994). Some argue that one of the most powerful forms of social control over women's sexuality is the fear of violence from men (Smart and Smart 1978).

Gender does not mean "sex" — although sex is determined by genes and biology, a gender perspective recognizes the socially defined, sexually differentiated roles and power relationships between women and men in society (Crawford and Maracek 1989; Balmer 1994; Cook 1994). Vlassoff (1994, p. 1249) explains "gender" as "the context of [the] behaviour [of women and men] in society, the different roles that they perform, the variety of social and cultural expectations and constraints placed upon them by

These biological differences, combined with intrapsychic processes and social learning, were believed to result in typical masculine and feminine characteristics. Typical masculine traits included strength, assertiveness, rationality, and biologically driven sex needs; whereas, feminine characteristics included softness, dependence, passivity, emotionality, and physical attractiveness.

— Anna Strebel, University of the Cape, Belleville, South Africa

virtue of their sex, and the ways they cope with societal expectations and constraints." Finally, Rathgeber (1994b, pp. 6–7) puts it this way:

Utilization of the term "gender" rather than "women" allows for a more substantive and profound analysis of the position of women vis-à-vis that of men .... Such an analysis will include a consideration of relations of power between men and women and inevitably it will lead to a questioning of basic social structures in a fundamental way.

Gender must be understood as a conditioning factor of all aspects of social life: in the work force, in the family, in political and cultural relations, as well as in ways of relating with the environment (Breilh 1994). Incorporating a gender perspective into health research is crucial if the research outputs are to lead to sustainable policy decisions.

It must also be emphasized that gender does not mean "woman." The subtitle of this book reflects the theme of most of the workshop presentations and discussions, which highlighted women's health issues. This focus on women reflects the need to "strengthen women and to redress imbalances in the power relations between women and men" (Richters 1994). In research and interventions aimed at improving the health of women, however, many participants stressed the importance of including men. In the area of sexually transmitted diseases (STD) and AIDS prevention, for example, men have much decision-making power in matters of sexuality and need to be encouraged to take the initiative for prevention. In the words of Barbara Klugman (1994), "there is increasing recognition in women's health circles [of the] need to research and address men's experiences and concerns given their power in relation to women." As well, in the distribution of childrearing and household responsibilities, men should also be persuaded to take a greater role to lessen the burden placed on women.

Gender stereotypes

Gender stereotypes are culturally shared expectations of gender-appropriate behaviours (Eagly and Steffen 1984; Eagly and Wood 1991; Garcia et al.

> As an individual grows, sex-linked attitudes and behaviours
> develop. Early in life, traits of passivity, dependency, and
> helplessness are established in women. In keeping with this
> gender-defined role, a woman or other family members may
> underplay her achievements to maintain the status quo.
>
> — S.A. Udipi and M.A. Varghese, SNDT Women's University, Bombay, India

1994). Although gender-role stereotypes change over time and vary from culture to culture, much of the control of women by men in our societies depends on these stereotypical roles. Gender-based social roles define the nature and type of activities pursued by women and men and define the power differential in male–female relationships (Airhihenbuwa et al. 1992; Garcia et al. 1994).

Traditional expectations of how males and females should behave can have severe consequences for the health and well-being of men, as well as women. Socialized expectations of men to be self-contained, emotionally controlled, and self-sufficient can lead to blocked emotions, a lack of openness, an inability to acknowledge weakness and vulnerability, and decreased capacity to receive interpersonal feedback (Pleck 1985; Werrbach and Gilbert 1987; Balmer 1994). Furthermore, "by centring maleness around a penile function and sexual prowess, society has nurtured an emotional atrophy in men that makes them all the more vulnerable to the dangers of risk-taking" (Pinel 1994, p. 67).

Women, on the other hand, are socialized in most cultures to be emotional, sensitive, nurturing, interdependent, and nonviolent, and such stereotypical expectations serve to stultify women.

Fluctuations in the nature of sexually defined roles throughout history and from society to society suggest that increased convergence in gender roles is possible (Balmer 1994). In the Philippines, for example, men and women inherit land equally. Where women have equal economic security to men, women also tend to have equal social and political power. Filipina women make up a significant proportion of the country's entrepreneurs, lawyers, and bank managers. Although women are expected to be quiet in many societies, Violeta Lopez-Gonzaga (1995) from the University of St La Salle (Bacolod) in the Philippines believes that it is culturally acceptable for women to talk as much as men in the Philippines and that there is no gender discrimination about a child's right to speak.

In Canada, an increasing number of women are entering traditionally male-dominated professions and more men are sharing household

"Marianismo," the feminine counterpart of "machismo," restricts women's values to virginity, motherhood, and her caretaking ability. The docile and submissive character of "marianismo" stimulates the existence of covert seduction, in opposition to assertiveness, as an almost exclusive way of meeting women's needs. Confrontation is not only considered improper, but is to be avoided, because it could invoke men's wrath. Women have been trapped into a disadvantageous, hierarchical structure that leaves them subject to discrimination, sexual harassment, and economical manipulation. It does not matter whether they are the primary caregivers or, in many cases, the main sources of family income, women's social vulnerability has superseded their abilities.

— Arletty Pinel, GENOS International, São Paulo, Brazil

responsibilities with their partners. Balmer (1994) argued that genuine equality between the sexes, which can greatly contribute to improved health for both women and men, will only be achieved with the breakdown of sharply differentiated gender stereotypes.

HEALTH

According to the widely recognized definition of health adopted by the WHO, health is a state of complete physical, mental, and social well-being and not merely the absence of disease or infirmity. The WHO concept of health "emphasizes the significance of the social welfare of populations and not merely the medicalization of disease" (Cook 1994, p. 5) and allows for the consideration of the complex set of cultural, economic, social, political, and environmental factors, as well as biological and genetic components, that influence the health and well-being of populations (Tsikata 1994). This broad definition acknowledges the role of human activities, social structures, and the environment in good health and creates the space to discuss the role of gender relations in health (Tsikata 1994).

To achieve a state of "complete physical, mental, and social well-being," a number of prerequisites for health have been identified by various commentators. To begin with, adequate shelter, nourishing food, good hygienic practices, clean and abundant water, and fuel are clearly essential. Health and well-being also requires peace, freedom from violence, access to income-earning capacity and opportunities, access to educational resources, social justice, a stable ecosystem, and sustainable resources (Cook 1994; Timoteo and Llanos-Cuentas 1994).

Actions undertaken outside the health sector can have much greater health effects than actions within the health sector. Therefore, to improve and sustain health, broad-based, intersectoral, and multisectoral activities at a number of levels are required to develop truly effective and integrative programs and policies (Milio 1986).

SUSTAINABLE DEVELOPMENT

In *Our Common Future*, the World Commission on Environment and Development states that to have development that is sustainable is to "ensure that it meets the needs of the present without compromising the ability of future generations to meet their own needs" (WCED 1987, p. 8). Healthy human beings are central to sustainable development. Investments in health can translate into healthier men, women, and children and increased capacity to lead socially and economically productive lives. Children who are healthy grow and learn better and have an improved chance of developing the skills necessary for employment. Incapacitation as a result of illness or the death of a household head can lead to family crisis and a vicious downward spiral of ill-health and poverty.

Women's health is a critical component of sustainable development. Although most of the world's poor suffer from poor health and nutrition, women often suffer from higher rates of malnutrition and greater burdens of illness and disability than men. Assuring women's good health means that they will be better able to perform their essential roles both inside and outside the home.

The correlation between health and sustainable development has often been overlooked because concepts of development have been traditionally associated with economic improvement. Development means more

Development must be concerned with enlarging people's choices for the realization of long and healthy lives; allowing people to achieve educational levels that will allow them to function adequately; and providing people with access to economic resources to allow for a decent standard of living.

— H. Elizabeth Thompson, Minister of Health, Barbados

*The results of the trickle-down economic growth paradigm that
has driven development programs since the 1960s as well as
the structural-adjustment programs that emerged in the 1980s
have seemingly brought about increased economic growth.
This, however, has come at a high price in terms of
the overall well-being of large proportions of the
populations of many developing nations.*

— Vivienne Wee, Centre for Environment, Gender and Development
(ENGENDER), Singapore

than economic growth alone. New models of development that invest in human potential and create enabling environments for the full use of human capabilities are needed. Development should focus directly on people and health as key variables and not be restricted to the increase of income and wealth.

Development that is sustainable must also be equitable. To date, however, women have been unequal beneficiaries of the forces of international development programs. In Gotarka, India, for example, despite the fact that a great deal of development money has been directed to ease the burden of the poor, women, who are the poorest of the poor, are the least likely to benefit. According to Stackhouse (1995a, p. D1):

> For all the fine intentions of outsiders, it is the men who tend to benefit from development — and the richer men at that. While women walk the dirt trails carrying headloads of wood, the wealthy men drive tractors on pukka roads. The men are paid high government wages for building water pipes; the women are expected to maintain these pipes for no wages at all. The schools are filled with male students. Even at the health centre, the ward is occupied by men because women will not allow a male practitioner to see their bodies uncovered.

Chapter 2

Crosscutting Issues

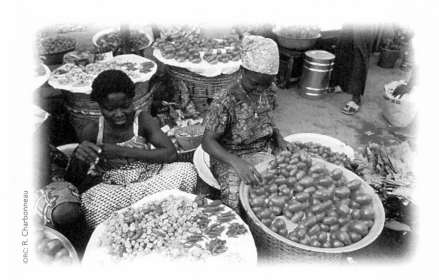

IDRC: R. Charbonneau

> *Where women have poor health status, it is a result of the*
> *different types of poverty from which they suffer. This refers*
> *not only to poverty in an economic sense, but to the*
> *multidimensional poverty that can start even before birth, when*
> *an infant girl is seen as a liability rather than an asset. It is the*
> *poverty that results when she is valued less, fed less, put to*
> *work at a very early age, denied schooling, and denied access*
> *to resources, technology, and essential services that respond to*
> *her health needs. This insidious poverty follows her throughout*
> *her entire life. These multifaceted and interlinking aspects of*
> *poverty ultimately determine health outcomes.*

— A. El Bindari Hammad, World Health Organization, Geneva, Switzerland

In the course of presentations and discussions that explored the four selected priority gender and health-research areas (AIDS, the working environment, tropical diseases, and barriers to quality health care), several themes emerged repeatedly. Four topics were identified as crosscutting issues that influence all aspects of women's health and well-being:

✦ The links between gender, class, and ethnicity;

✦ The correlation between women's education and health;

✦ The relationship between the empowerment of women and health; and

✦ The role of nutrition.

GENDER, CLASS, AND ETHNICITY

There is a growing recognition that class and race variables intersect with gender to compound the complexity of power relations (Ramazanoglu 1989; Stamp 1989; Singer 1994; Strebel 1994). Disadvantaged racial groups in rich countries are often in worse health that better-off groups living in poor countries. The health status of Canadian Indians, for example, lags far behind the general Canadian population. The maternal mortality rate for the registered Indian population was, on average, five times the Canadian rate between 1984 and 1988. In 1988, the Indian infant mortality rate was 2.2 times the Canadian rate (Health and Welfare Canada 1991). And, in the United States, "the intersection of urban poverty and socially devalued ethnicity (especially being African-American and Latino, and in some parts of the country Native American and Asian as well) have proven to be a particularly unhealthy combination" (Singer 1994, p. 931).

A number of interrelated conditions, disproportionately affecting poor African-American and Latino women and men, have led to the health crises in inner cities of America. These include high rates of unemployment, homelessness, residential overcrowding, substandard nutrition, environmental toxins, infrastructural deterioration, forced geographic mobility, family breakup, disruption of social-support networks, youth-gang and drug-related violence, and health-care inequalities (Singer 1994). Although the United States, and to a lesser extent Canada, provide graphic examples of the sharp socioeconomic and health-related differences that exist depending on race and class, these types of disparities can be found in most countries of the world.

An intersectoral approach must therefore be adopted when addressing health issues. The approach must link gender as a system of inequity with other forms of inequity such as class and ethnicity (Breilh 1994). This type of approach may help to explain why men in Bangladesh have a higher probability of survival after age 35 than men in Harlem, New York (McCord and Freeman 1990).

Just as health issues for men are different from those faced by women, diseases of the rich are not the same as diseases of the poor. As remarked by Vivienne Wee: "Poor black women living in the United States are among the worst off. On all three levels — race, class, and gender — they are the poorest of the poor." And as echoed by Rosina Wiltshire: "Although there are inequalities related to race and class, it is important to focus on gender ... women suffer most regardless of race or class."

The role of poverty

The majority of the world's poor are women. Women often lack power and social status in society and, therefore, access to economic resources (Strebel 1994). As a result of their differential positioning in society, women are usually poorer than men, and are often economically dependent on men (Campbell 1990; Ankrah 1991; Ulin 1992).

It is impossible to talk about the feminization of poverty without mentioning the increasing number of single women with children who are heads of households. This worldwide phenomenon is the result of national and international migration of men in the search for work, divorce, widowhood, wars, desertion, and the increasing number of births to unpartnered adolescent women. Female-headed households, which make up about one-quarter of households around the world (UN 1995), are particularly disadvantaged and economically vulnerable. The lack of educational opportunities for

Pigsties are better than many of the shacks of these people here. It is difficult to have self-esteem that way, everything points to your undervaluation as a person. They do not take care of themselves as people, they belittle themselves as women, they have no self-respect.

— A health professional commenting on the lives of women living in extreme poverty outside Montevideo, Uruguay, reported by Maria Bonino, Universidad de la República, Montevideo, Uruguay

women and the difficulties obtaining well-paid secure employment mean that the amount of money coming into female-headed households is usually considerably less than into male-headed households (Acevedo 1994). As explained by Richters (1994, p. 41): "Because such mothers are often poorly educated, without investment capital, and attempt to do two jobs at once (domestic and wage work), female-headed households tend to be poor."

Poverty has a powerful influence on health. Female poverty means that less money is available to purchase adequate and nutritious foods, which increases the risk of illness and disease. Inadequate nutrition influences disease recovery. Substandard living conditions, including poor housing, deficient standards of hygiene, unhealthy sources of water, and lack of garbage collection services and sewage systems, also expose populations to increased risk of disease. Poor women are also unlikely to have access to formal health-care services and adequate treatment and tend to give birth to babies of low birth weight who begin life in a disadvantaged state.

Poverty affects a woman's available life choices. Female poverty can mean that a woman has to take whatever job she can get to support herself and her family; this lack of choice greatly increases the probability that she will end up working in an exploitative situation with little or no occupational health and safety protection. Entering into prostitution is another strategy used by women around the world to cope with poverty.

Harsh living conditions can also lead to feelings of negativity and low self-esteem, which are important psychological variables affecting the attitudes of women about their health. Poor self-esteem and self-respect reduce the likelihood that a woman will seek out health-care services for her own needs.

Policies aimed at increasing the economic opportunities of women living in poverty will ultimately improve the health and well-being of women, as well as other household members. Women usually spend additional income on ways that enhance their health — improving their diet, obtaining safe water, and upgrading sanitation and housing. "In the developing world, women tend to spend whatever wealth they have on food, education, and health care for their children, whereas men tend to spend on such things as prestige goods, alcohol and extra-marital sexual liaisons" (Richters 1994, p. 40)

WOMEN'S EDUCATION AND HEALTH

A second crosscutting issue influencing women's health and well-being concerns the correlation between the education of women and health. In almost all developing countries, women are disadvantaged as a result of poorer educational opportunities. According to the *Report of the International Conference on Population and Development*, which was held 5–13 September 1994 in Cairo (UN 1994):

> There are approximately 960 million illiterate adults in the world, of whom two thirds are women. More than one third of the world's adults, most of them women, have no access to printed knowledge, to new skills or to technologies that would improve the quality of their lives .... There are 130 million children who are not enrolled in primary school and 70 per cent of them are girls.

In Viet Nam, "high rates of school dropout among girls are an indication of both high education expenses and the lack of emphasis placed on female education" (Binh 1995). In India, no more than 33% of girls receive a minimal 5 000 hours of schooling, or about 6 full years; whereas, in China and Latin America, only 60% of girls receive this minimal level of education (World Bank 1993). Women's rates of enrollment in secondary schools lag behind men's by as much as 56% in Bangladesh, 40% in Malawi, and 68% in Togo (Misch 1992). Although some countries have been able to achieve gender equity in enrollment rates at primary schools (Tillett 1994), the higher the education level, the more likely that gender gaps prevail, particularly at the tertiary level (Grandea 1994).

Female education, gender–power relations, and AIDS must be considered not only separately, but also as dynamically interconnected.

— Maureen Law, International Development Research Centre, Ottawa, Canada (see Law 1994)

Reduced access to education, information, and knowledge means that women are often poorly informed about health issues, about how their bodies function, and about how to protect themselves from disease, and disadvantaged in their ability to recognize and act on signs and symptoms of illness (Manderson 1994; Vlassoff 1994). Poverty of education "creates a vicious circle of myth and misinformation that perpetuates health-damaging behaviours and harmful practices" (Hammad 1994, p. 3).

The call for better educational opportunities for women is often premised on the fact that educated women are better mothers, who raise fewer, better educated, and healthier children (Grandea 1994). As the World Bank (1993, p. 42) pointed out:

> In developing countries better-educated women marry and start their families later .... Educated women also tend to make greater use of pre-natal care and delivery assistance ... the children of educated mothers continue to enjoy other health-enhancing advantages: better domestic hygiene, which reduces the risk of infection; better food and more immunization, both of which reduce susceptibility to infection; and wiser use of medial services ... slower population growth and lower infant morality rates are closely associated with increasing levels of women's education.

However, greater education for women not only means that their children will be healthier, it also means that women themselves will be healthier. Education "increases [women's] ability to benefit from health information and to make good use of health services; it increases their access to income and enables them to live healthier lives" (World Bank 1993, p. 42). For example, Mbacke and van de Walle (1987) found that the use of mosquito nets and coils was significantly related to maternal education. Education also instills confidence in women to deal with the world.

It is a well-documented fact that educated women visit their health providers more often than uneducated women as education increases self-respect and self-confidence in women. Educated women also have more knowledge of the health-care system. The effect of education extends beyond her to the attitudes of others around her, including health providers who will treat her with more respect and consideration. Education improves communication between the female client and the health provider. As a result, the educated woman's experience with the health provider may be more favourable than that of the uneducated woman.

— Tehseen Iqbal, Multan, Pakistan

Women with higher levels of formal and nonformal education may have greater family decision-making power on health and related matters (Sermsri 1995). Energy intake of girls in a slum community outside Bombay, India, was found to be positively and significantly influenced by educational status and decision-making power (Udipi and Varghese 1995). A study conducted in rural southern India found that mothers who had been to school were more likely to demand of their husbands and mothers-in-law that a sick child be treated and more likely to use medical facilities. They were also more likely to follow the doctor's instructions and return to the health centre for further care (Caldwell 1993).

Educated women and mothers may have greater decision-making power on health and related matters within both the family and the community, be more knowledgeable about disease prevention and treatment, and be more likely to adopt new codes of behaviour that improve the health of their children.

— Santhat Sermsri, International Forum for Social Sciences in Health, Nakornpathom, Thailand

Women's opportunities in the work force, and the possibility of obtaining jobs that provide adequate wages[2] are at least partially linked to education. Education is an important factor underlying gender segregation in the labour market. Women's training tends to be oriented toward particular career paths, such as those in the social sector, such as teaching, nursing, and typing, and away from technical or industrial fields (ILO 1985; Grandea 1994). Unless gender-based inequities in education are removed, women will not have the basic prerequisites to compete for high-skilled, high-paying jobs (Grandea 1994).

Although education can, to some extent, increase the possibility of women obtaining better jobs, the link between eduction and employment, particularly for women, is fragile. Even when women have the right skills, gender stereotypes and cultural dictates, as well as socioeconomic factors, can present barriers to equal opportunity for women (Grandea 1994).

In some societies, parents are reluctant to invest in the education of girls and do not encourage their daughters to remain in school (Atai-Okei 1994; Kerawalla 1994). In an urban slum outside Bombay, India, Muslim families said that girls should not be educated because education causes them

---

[2] Sufficient to afford nutritious and adequate food and proper accommodations with healthy sources of water and an environmentally safe power supply.

to be more vocal, independent, and autonomous and leads them to "talk back" to their elders (Udipi and Varghese 1995). Other reasons why parents keep their daughters out of school include "fear of too much freedom ... a preference for increasing limited resources in their sons' education with a view to parental support in old age ... better job prospects and wage rates for men [and] traditional stereotypes of women's roles" (UN 1995, p. 91).

> Investing in the education of children has traditionally been seen as a loan to be repaid by children. Daughters are educated so that they can return much of the "investment" before marriage. They are sent out to work as soon as possible so they can contribute to the family economy, including the education of their siblings, especially their brothers. Although the education of daughters is expected to help the marriage alliance, education of daughters as a value in itself has had very little recognition.
>
> — S.A. Udipi and M.A. Varghese, SNDT Women's University, Bombay, India

The link between education and improved health may be correlated to higher income levels — indeed, income may be the determining factor. Better-off families can afford to send their girls to school longer and may be more inclined to consider the education of children to be an investment for the future. In poor families, however, demanding household duties often result in children getting taken out of school to work. Young girls, especially, drop out of school to help their mothers. When a mother becomes seriously ill, her daughter is more likely than her son to be kept from schooling to assume increased domestic responsibilities.

Policies to expand schooling for girls are crucial to promote health. Educational facilities must be created and strengthened and girls must be provided the same opportunity for education as boys. Essential health information should be introduced into school curricula at the earliest levels.

EMPOWERMENT OF WOMEN AND HEALTH

The links between women's health and notions of empowerment, entitlement, and improved self-esteem formed another crosscutting issue. "Empowerment" literally means the investing of power and authority. The word has come to mean enabling or equipping individuals or groups to have power, with the aim of creating and fostering relationships of equals in society. "For women, the process of empowerment entails breaking away from

Once a woman has self-esteem she begins to "find the person within the woman," and starts to take responsibility for her own health needs.

— S.A. Udipi and M.A. Varghese, SNDT Women's University, Bombay, India

the cycle of learned and taught submission to discrimination, carried from one generation of women to the next" (Tomasevski 1993, p. 24). Nan Peacocke (1995), from the Women and Development Unit (WAND) of the University of the West Indies, believes that a sense of empowerment is critical to get women to accept health-related information and translate this knowledge into behavioural changes.

The widespread devaluation of women in society can be seen in the relative lack of educational opportunities for women and the unequal allocation of resources to women, such as land and food. Women's interests are undermined, and their work is devalued. The general low status of women, and their internalization of this status, results in the marginalization of women's physical, psychological, and emotional needs (Kwawu 1994; Manderson 1994). As stated by Lin Tan (1995): "Women's position in society directly or indirectly influences their ability to participate in childbearing, sexual conduct, and fertility-rate decisions."

Increased understanding by women of their value in the family and the community and the important contribution their labour makes to the national economy can lead to increased confidence and self-esteem, can affect women's interactions with others, and can lead to positive changes in health behaviour (Peacocke 1995). When a woman's self-esteem improves, increasingly she feels able to make more household decisions and begin to put forward her viewpoints within the family.

The formation of women's groups can lead to increased self-confidence and self-esteem on the part of women (Udipi and Varghese 1995). A women's group, formed in a slum community outside Bombay, India, where the mobility of women was significantly curtailed, provided women with the opportunity to come out of the household as a first step and gradually led them to take the initiative to improve their own health and well-being. The formation of another group in Surkhet, Nepal, helped women to talk openly about their problems and encouraged them to gradually break down traditional discriminatory practices that work against women's health. One women announced after giving birth that she would set her own diet, complete with vegetables; whereas, other women "have begun to quietly tuck away one handful of rice a day to eat later or to sell" (Stackhouse 1995b, p. A7).

> *In the beginning, women would be absorbed in household affairs and often said they had no time to participate. When some of us got together and started a preschool centre and skill-training program, women became curious. Today we have many women who find that they can manage their household activities and tasks better and spare 2 or 3 hours. More importantly, they feel this spare time is to be devoted to themselves. The [women's group] has gradually helped women to voice their inner feelings first in the group and then [they are better able] to speak within the family.*
>
> — A community worker, quoted by S.A. Udipi and M.A. Varghese,
> SNDT Women's University, Bombay, India

Women must be encouraged to take control over their own health: "The notions of self-care, and control over one's life, need to be felt at every emotional level" (Pinel 1994, p. 57). Furthermore, women must be taught skills that enable them to effectively change their reality.

Finally, a sense of entitlement can make it possible for women to challenge existing power structures. As an illustration, Peacocke (1995, pp. 278–279) described how one woman, C.J., a member of the Red Thread Women's Development Organization in Guyana, was able to effect change at a workshop on breastfeeding because of her sense of entitlement and her understanding of the sociocultural determinants of health. C.J. provided the following account of her experiences:

> I went to a workshop on Thursday and Friday. When I get there I said to myself, "What! [Why did the team leader] send me here?" It was sheer doctors, sheer "up there!" When we [got] into small group discussion I had to tell the doctor who was the facilitator, "I think we [are] starting wrong ... let us look at the chronic diseases first." [C.J. explained that the doctor looked surprised that an alternative approach was offered, while the nurses were shocked that C.J. had contradicted a doctor]. I tell you 20 minutes and they can't start yet! Then, you know what the doctor say? "OK, let's start how C.J. said we should." You know, when we started we had a smooth flow of discussion.
>
> In my evaluation I said, "You know what? I personally feel this workshop here hasn't achieved its aim. We ... needed more grassroots people at this workshop, because the grassroots people could tell you ... doctors and nurses about breastfeeding and tell you why they are not breastfeeding babies." One of the decisions they came up with [was] that they are going to give mothers 4 months maternity leave so they could breastfeed babies. I said, "That 4 months still can't do anything because the mothers ain't getting proper food to eat."

NUTRITION

Women's nutrition is another crosscutting issue that influences all aspects of women's health and well-being. Although the nutritional status of women has received significant attention in research and interventions addressing women's health, "in most cases the primary objective has been the improvement of infant nutritional status ... very little attention has been paid to the problem of nutritional deficiencies among non-pregnant, non-lactating women" (Paolisso and Leslie 1995, p. 57).

Women suffer disproportionately from iron-deficiency anemia, iodine-deficiency disorders, and from stunting caused by protein–energy malnutrition (Figure 1). Throughout the world, 43% of women and 51% of pregnant women suffer from iron-deficiency anemia. Pregnancy puts a severe strain on women's iron status and 56% of pregnant women in developing countries are anemic (rising to 88% in India) (WHO 1994b). Anemia is also a risk for non-pregnant women because of the iron demand of lactation and the iron losses associated with menstruation (Paolisso and Leslie 1995).

Women's nutritional status can be significantly affected by the unequal distribution of food among family members, which is linked to women's lower social status (Breilh 1994; Rathgeber 1994a). Discrimination can begin in early infancy with male children being breastfed longer than girl children (Udipi and Varghese 1995). In some regions of the world, men and boys routinely eat first, and women and girls "eat less food which is of inferior quality and nutritive value" (UN 1991).

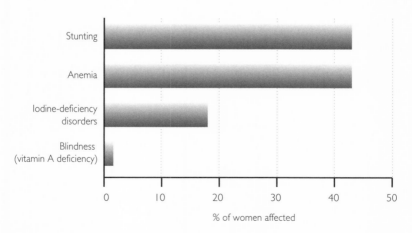

Figure 1. Percentage of women (15 years and above) who are affected by stunting, anemia, iodine-deficiency disorders, and blindness from vitamin A deficiency (1992) (source: WHO 1994b).

Discriminatory feeding practices in childhood can lead to protein–energy deficiency. The stunting that results in the girl may cause problems in her subsequent reproductive life such as obstructed labour, birth asphyxia, and many other conditions.

— A. El Bindari Hammad, World Health Organization, Geneva, Switzerland

A survey in India by the National Committee on the Status of Women found that women ate after men in 48.5% of households (Udipi and Varghese 1995). Mothers "drill[ed] the sacrificial role into daughters with regard to food intake" (Udipi and Varghese 1995, p. 154). Male family members who ate first did not think about whether the amount of food available was sufficient for the whole family and were insensitive to the nutritional needs of female family members (Udipi and Varghese 1995).

Food deprivation is part of the socialization of girls; it is seen as part of their deferential role that they will continue to play as future daughters-in-law. Parents often explain that discrimination against girl children is part of their training, so that they will know what is expected of them in the homes of their in-laws.

— S.A. Udipi and M.A. Varghese, SNDT Women's University, Bombay, India

Research in the Philippines (Illo 1991, p. 4) has also shown that women tend to place themselves last when serving food among their family members.

> The male spouse's food has to be secured first, then the children's. This is particularly true during lean months when rice and other food are scarce, and some rationing occurs ... many of the women ... interviewed seemed to consider this abstinence as part of being a good wife and mother.

Selected health effects of inadequate nutrition

Inadequate nourishment limits the physical development of women, compromises their health, and threatens their ability to bear healthy children. "Malnourished women are sick more, have smaller babies, and die earlier" (UN 1991).

✦ *Nutrition and AIDS:* Women frequently have a poorer prognosis once infected with HIV and die sooner than men (Jones and Catalan 1989; Berer and Ray 1993; Melnick et al. 1994; Strebel 1994). This may be related to the fact that the progression of AIDS is associated with the basic health and immune status of the individual prior to infection, and women tend to have poor general health and nutrition (Adeokun 1994).

✦ *Nutrition and women's work:* Nutritional anemia exacerbates fatigue and reduces the working capacity of women in the workplace and at home (UN 1991). Poor nutrition may also increase the effects of workplace illness (Haile 1994; Puta 1994). As Messing (1991, p. 10) pointed out: "The healthy young body may resist damage from workplace chemicals better than the unhealthy or older body ... the poorly nourished body may be less able to tolerate polluted air."

✦ *Nutrition and tropical diseases:* Inadequate nutrition compromises the immunological status of women and enhances their susceptibility to tropical diseases (Ulrich et al. 1992). The depressed health status of women as a result of general malnutrition has been identified as one of the reasons for high levels of mortality and morbidity in women from malaria (Alilio 1994). A synergism between nutrition and visceral leishmaniasis has also been reported, and children with signs of malnutrition are more likely to get this disease (Mutinga 1984).

✦ *Nutrition and barriers to quality health care:* Poorly nourished women are less likely to pay attention to health-education messages essential to their own health (Alilio 1994). Not only are poorly nourished women less likely to attend to their own health needs, they may also feel less inclined to participate in activities such as attending prenatal care and taking their children for growth-monitoring and immunization (Alilio 1994).

Hypertension, diabetes, and obesity among Caribbean women

Researchers from the Caribbean highlighted that poor nutrition among Caribbean women coexists with a high susceptibility to nutrition-related diseases such as hypertension, diabetes, and obesity. Indeed, these diseases are among the main causes of death among women in the Caribbean (Patterson 1995). Furthermore, the prevalence of such diseases is several times higher in women than in men (Fraser 1995; Patterson 1995; Thompson 1995).

The presence of these diseases may be related to an imbalance in the nutrient content of the food consumed within households (Patterson 1995). Cultural practices that emphasize the use of salt, simple sugars, and fats in the diet may be partially responsible. Importance continues to be placed on calorie-rich foods, historically a necessity, but no longer relevant in more modern societies. Indigenous foods, rich in complex carbohydrates, fibre, beta carotenes, and other vitamins, are rejected by some segments of the population as "poor people's food" (Patterson 1995). Avenues to change these traditional and cultural perceptions are essential in the management of these diseases.

Fraser (1995) pointed out that high female susceptibility to obesity is also related to the fact that obesity in Caribbean women has traditionally been regarded as a sign of beauty and good health. Women who are thin, even if they are healthy, may be considered to be ill. However, recent evidence has suggested that, at least among the younger generation, these attitudes may be changing (Fraser 1995).

Finally, some research studies in North America have demonstrated a relationship between cardiovascular disease and poverty and social inequality (Singer 1994). These links needs to be explored, particularly from a Caribbean context.

Environmental degradation and nutrition

In Chapter 6, the impact of environmental degradation on women's work is addressed. Environmental degradation not only increases the workloads of women, it can also lead to difficulties for community members in meeting their nutritional needs. In the Tongu area of Ghana, for example, environmental degradation has led to the loss of clams and the deterioration of

The lack of food places great stress on women who are usually the food providers. They can no longer produce their own carbohydrates and protein. Most food now has to be imported from the Afram plains and other parts of the country to be sold in Tongu communities. Low incomes make it difficult to afford enough food, especially proteins, which are expensive. This situation has significantly contributed to high levels of anemia and malnutrition, as well as reduced resistance to other diseases.

— Dzodzi Tsikata, Institute of Statistical, Social and Economic Research, University of Ghana, Legon, Ghana

fishing and farming, which has drastically affected nutritional standards (Tsikata 1994). Lack of food is now one of the most serious problems in this area; community members must buy foods that they once produced, which is particularly difficult for low-income families.

Jacobson (1992a, p. 26) reported that deforestation, and the "scarcity of leaves, twigs, branches, grasses, and other materials used for cooking fuel now rivals the scarcity of food itself as a cause of malnutrition in parts of sub-Saharan Africa, Haiti, Mexico, Nepal, and Thailand." Without wood "women cannot cook the food they have grown and harvested, or do simple things like boil water or heat their homes." With less fuelwood available, women may either cook meals for less time or reduce the number of cooked meals, which leads to undernutrition.

In some parts of the world, agricultural fields have been ravaged by war and this has led to poor levels of nutrition in affected communities. In Cambodia, for example, the use of chemicals and land mines has adversely affected crop growth and therefore nutritional levels (Ren et al. 1995). Women, primarily responsible for feeding their families, feel the effects of these food shortages most acutely.

Crops do not produce as much as before because they have to be sown time and time again to yield enough for sale; the soil grows tired — and so do we.

— Quoted by Xochitl Herrera and Miguel Lobo-Guerrero, Etnollano Foundation, Bogotá, Colombia

Replacement of indigenous subsistence-farming activities with income-generation activities may lead to a deterioration of community nutritional standards and of the ecology of the land. For example, among indigenous communities in the Orinoco and Amazon basins of South America, an intensification of commercial relations with the nonindigenous world has caused many alterations to traditional society. Traditionally, each indigenous family usually has two or three *conucos* (plots of land) where they grow a wide variety of crops for home consumption, such as pineapple, *mapuey*, yucca, peppers, *seje*, and *lulo* (Herrera and Lobo-Guerrera 1994). Together, these crops constituted a balanced diet and maintained the quality of the soil (Rojas 1992). However, as indigenous subsistence agricultural societies increasingly turn to income-generation activities, traditional *conucos* have become dedicated to the planting of a single commercial crop, such as cocoa, bananas, maize, or yucca. A "good" *conuco* now means "a big *conuco*, full of bananas," instead of a diverse plot growing a variety of nutritious foods for family consumption. This can have long-term effects on the nutritional levels of the community because the soil used for crops in the Orinoco basin, like the soil used in the Amazon rain forests, is fragile and will not bear intensive commercial cultivation.

Chapter 3

The Research Process

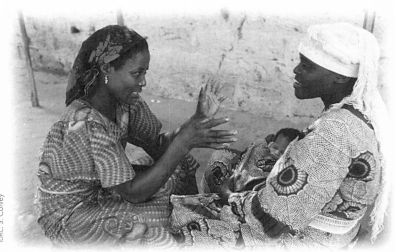

> The health needs of women, and the constraints to
> meeting those needs, take a heavy toll on women. Most
> could be prevented or substantially reduced, however,
> through improved interventions based on more
> comprehensive, gender-disaggregated,
> interdisciplinary research.
>
> — Michael Paolisso and Joanne Leslie, International Centre for Research on
> Women, Washington, DC, USA (see Paolisso and Leslie 1995, p. 62)

BARRIERS TO RESEARCH

Various obstacles hinder the adoption of a gender perspective in health research. There is sometimes a lack of institutional and financial support for gender and health research, and many researchers lack the necessary research tools. In some cases, recent publications, good research, and bibliographies are difficult to access. In Latin America, researchers have difficulty obtaining resources in the Spanish language. The dearth of health research that incorporates a gender perspective, for example, in tropical disease research and the study of occupational health and safety, represents another barrier to research. There is also a need for in-depth training with regard to methodologies, techniques, and specific instruments for studying gender dimensions and for some form of a "checklist" that could be followed to ensure that research is gender-sensitive.

Beyond these barriers, it can take great efforts to overcome a "masculine-oriented perspective" (Lange et al. 1994). For example, Ilta Lange, in her research on health monitors in Santiago, Chile, found that masculine language dominated the research process. The Spanish word "monitores" was always used, instead of "monitoras," the feminine version of the word. Although all the health monitors studied were women, Lange said researchers persisted in using the masculine form of the word.

Finally, community resistance to certain types of research can also be an obstacle. Pino et al. (1994) reported that parents and teachers in Santiago, Chile, tried to prevent research that involved the study of adolescents and early sexual behaviour. Such barriers must be overcome. Research in this area is needed to help design sound programs and policies aimed at reducing the number of unwanted pregnancies and the incidence of sexually transmitted diseases, including AIDS, among adolescents.

A GENDER PERSPECTIVE

A gender perspective cannot simply be added to a study as an afterthought. It must be fully integrated into the research protocol as it is conceived, carried out, analyzed, and disseminated. A gender perspective also involves much more than sex disaggregation. At the very least, however, "sex should be a variable taken into account in ... studies, even where understanding sex differences as such are not inherent to the study objectives" (Vlassoff 1994, p. 1256). The existing lack of sex-disaggregated data and information hinders the ability of decision-makers to develop effective women's health programs and policies.

In addition to providing information on the sex of respondents and why they were selected, studies should furnish information "on the social structural and cultural context in the society under investigation" (Vlassoff 1994, p. 1257). Ideally, health research should address differential female and male roles; responsibilities; knowledge bases; positions and status within society; attitudes and perception; access to and use of resources and information; and participation in decision-making; as well as social codes and attitudes governing female and male behaviour.

Because women and men often have different roles and responsibilities, their "environmental life spaces" within and outside the home can be quite different. The impact of these differing environments on health should be addressed.

Interdisciplinary research teams, which, for example, include researchers with medical backgrounds and social scientists, may facilitate the adoption of a gender perspective. It is impossible for any single discipline or type of specialist to "have the requisite expertise to identify the critical socio-biomedical factors determining women's health risks and needs" (Paolisso and Leslie 1995, p. 55). However, interdisciplinary teams are not always feasible because of insufficient resources. Because of this constraint, cross-disciplinary training, for example, highlighting social science issues and techniques in the medical school curriculum, and vice versa, is

---

The challenge is to find ways of ensuring that health studies are designed to take into account all the determinants of health and disease in any society so that gender differentials become visible to policymakers.

— Dzodzi Tsikata, Institute of Statistical, Social and Economic Research, University of Ghana, Legon, Ghana

> *Where does a man or a woman, a girl or a boy, a female baby or*
> *a male baby, stand 24 hours of the day? Men's and women's life*
> *spaces are different and this may lead to differential exposure to*
> *diseases and illnesses, including tropical diseases. This is tied to*
> *the gender division of labour. For example, who does the animal*
> *herding? Who picks up the cow dung? Who slaughters the animals?*
> *Who cleans the clothes and utensils in the river? Researchers*
> *could look at how many hours members of the population being*
> *studied spend each day at the office, in the field, at home, and so*
> *on. How often is the population exposed to certain hazards? If the*
> *community lives near a toxic waste dump, which community*
> *members — men, women, or children — are at home*
> *all day and most exposed to the dump?*
>
> — Vivienne Wee, Centre for Environment, Gender and Development
> (ENGENDER), Singapore

increasingly being carried out. However, researchers with scientific and medical backgrounds, even without social science training, can learn to look at their data from a new perspective. As human beings, medical researchers can uncover the human dimension and carry out social science research.

Having a gender perspective means being aware of, and accounting for, the plethora of gender-related factors that may affect the collection of research data. Researchers should be aware, for example, that women may have different notions of health and illness than men. Women, and in particular, poor women, may take a certain amount of aches and pain for granted. They may not report backaches as a health problem because they have a high threshold of pain, and view them as normal. "Women tend to suffer in silence ... the threshold of illness recognized by the society on the illness–health continuum is so high for women that they endure so much in order not to disrupt household organization" (Okojie 1994, p. 1237).

It may be extremely difficult for researchers to gather information that reflects the true state of affairs for women because, in some cultures, women may be reticent to speak their minds, particularly if men are around. Male heads of households may wish to speak "on behalf of women," even about subject matters that are particularly important to women. Researchers therefore need to ensure that women are able to speak for themselves. As Irene Luppi (1994) reported: "[With] the presence of husbands during the interviews, ... interviewers had to [cope with] the difficulties such presence presented when, for example, the husband would correct or censor the interviewee's answers, or would ask the interviewer to erase some answers, or would [say] that 'It'd be better that I answer cos' I know better.'"

The sex of the researcher is another important issue to be considered. In some societies, women are forbidden to open their doors to unknown males and this could result in the systematic skipping of women (Manderson 1994). Even if a male researcher is able to access both sexes, girls and women can feel uncomfortable being interviewed by a man and may resist answering his questions. They may feel greater ease expressing themselves with other women, particular concerning sensitive issues like sexuality. In her study of women and AIDS, Strebel (1993) reported that the use of female researchers helped to create a sense of shared experience, especially related to sexual matters and men's treatment of women. For evaluative purposes, study reports should be sure to identify whether the research team was made up of men, women, or a combination of both sexes.

The timing of interviews must also build in an appreciation of gender differences. Respondents may or may not be available to be interviewed given gender-differentiated roles and responsibilities. For example, in an agricultural community, the sample is likely to be skewed if interviews are conducted when most women are at work in the fields.

Participatory research methods are increasingly gaining acceptance and respect, and those methods tend to have a more feminist perspective because they tend to value everyone's opinion and give opportunity for everyone to speak.

— Eva M. Rathgeber, International Development Research Centre, Regional Office for Eastern and Southern Africa, Nairobi, Kenya

---

A potential methodological problem relates to the possible discrepancies between what women say they do, and what they actually do. For example, although women may be aware of what they should be doing to stay healthy, for various reasons, they may be unable to carry out desired health practices. If an interviewer asks, "what do you do when ...?" women may report what they believe is "the right answer" (that is, what they should be doing, not what they actually do). When looking at household nutritional practices, for example, women, as the designated "family caregivers," could be embarrassed to tell researchers about the difficulties they have in providing their children with nutritious and adequate foods. Researchers therefore need to find ways to learn about the gap between desired intentions and actual practices. It may be helpful to ask questions such as: "What are the difficulties that you face in carrying out what you know should be done?"

In the area of sexuality, women may be reluctant to be truthful with interviewers because of socialized gender expectations. When researching adolescent sexual activity, for example, the extent to which a respondent is truthful about this subject matter is related to the social acceptability of her or his conduct, which is largely conditioned by gender. Even if researchers take all steps necessary to ensure confidentiality and anonymity, results may still be affected by gender-differentiated societal expectations concerning premarital sex.

Researchers should ensure that the research topic is of concern to the community being studied. Women's voices need to be heard. Perspectives of women from the community should be included throughout the research process — community women should be involved in defining priorities for research, creating ethical guidelines and standards, creating and implementing the research design, and analyzing the results. Researchers from the Health Research and Consultancy Centre in Ecuador, for example, followed a model of participatory research in which the women helped administer questionnaires about their living and working conditions, health problems, and access to health care (Breilh 1994). Researchers should also be sensitive to the demands they place on women and ensure that the women are properly compensated for their time and efforts. To learn more about women's health needs, researchers can also draw on the expertise of groups who work closely with women and are likely to represent women's perspectives.

At the end of each focus group discussion, women spoke about how marvellous it was to have the opportunity to talk about issues that are usually ignored. After each discussion we gave the women information and answers to questions that had arisen during the discussion. This gave them useful knowledge and dealt with many of their anxieties. We promised to come back to them when we finished the research so that they could hear what other women had to say. Women expressed delight at this opportunity because they are so removed from the experiences of other women. This example illustrates how the research process can be enjoyable and beneficial to the "researched."

— Barbara Klugman, Women's Health Project, University of Witwatersrand, Johannesburg, South Africa (see Klugman 1994)

The researched population should also be fully informed of the results of the research. Women who participate in research should emerge from that interaction more conscious of their world and, thus, better able to act upon it (Klugman 1994). Many researchers in the past have exploited community members without giving back to the community. As remarked by Violeta Lopez-Gonzaga: "Many have received their PhD and reaped honours because of the time and labour sacrificed by community members, without empowering the people being studied." Strebel (1993) noted, however, that attempts to provide results to research participants were not always successful. She asserts that creative ways are needed to get research findings to connect with the immediate needs of participants.

QUALITATIVE RESEARCH

Many commentators have emphasized the importance of qualitative research techniques — such as key informants, focus-group discussions, and in-depth interviews — to provide a multidimensional view of social situations. In *Women in Development: Perspectives from the Nairobi Conference*, Ellis (1986, p. 138) comments:

> The qualitative approach helps us to understand people as they interact in various social contexts and to define social reality from their own experience, perspective and meaning rather than from that of the researcher alone .... It raises hitherto unasked questions, the answers to which afford deeper and sharper insights into how and why people participate as they do in a variety of social processes.

Also, according to Simmons and Elias (1994, p. 6):

> Qualitative methods, using primarily observational techniques and a variety of in-depth interviewing approaches, produce contextual or holistic explanations for a smaller number of cases, with an emphasis on meaning rather than the frequency of social phenomena.

Chiarella (1994) outlined five advantages of qualitative research: it is flexible, and allows for the development of the concept and model throughout the investigation; the data gathered need not always prove preconceived hypotheses or theories; it provides the possibility of investigating essential elements and people as a whole, not as variables; it rejects pre-established prejudices and beliefs and attempts to see facts or processes as if they were occurring for the first time; and the integration of data can be carried out from the point of view of the informants themselves. This last point is important because the way people talk about their lives is significant. "The language they use and the connections they make reveal the world that they see and in which they act" (Gilligan 1982, p. 2).

Several researchers have reported fascinating research results stemming from qualitative methods. Chiarella (1994), for example, obtained a wealth of qualitative information concerning why some indigenous women in Bolivia were reluctant to use western-based health-care services. Through qualitative techniques, researchers from Myanmar identified traditional customs and cultural beliefs toward pregnancy, explored the perceptions of married couples about pregnancy, and investigated the advantages and disadvantages of antenatal care (Win May et al. 1995). A study of the psychosocial determinants that influence the use of maternal and child-health services in areas of extreme poverty in Montevideo, Uruguay, had an initial qualitative stage aimed at learning more about the variables, indicators, and categories associated with the use or nonuse of health services (Bonino 1994). Individual and collective interviews were held with women in the area, as well as with health personnel, and a rich collection of information was gathered that would not have been obtained through quantitative methods.

Focus groups have many advantages. To begin with, focus groups can serve to reduce the potential power differential that may occur in one-on-one interviews. Focus groups, which have more participants than facilitators, allow conversations or discussions to occur among participants with only occasional direction from the facilitator. The facilitator, in effect, moves into the background, and any perceived difference in status or power between participants and the facilitator tends to be minimized. Focus groups can also serve to bring women together who share similar day-to-day life experiences. In the process of sharing their stories, the women themselves probe, challenge, and share information in greater depth than can usually be fostered in a single interview.

— Thicumporn Kuyyakanond, Northeast Centre for AIDS Prevention and Care, Khon Kaen University, Thailand

---

The research question should determine whether qualitative or quantitative techniques, or a combination of both approaches, are used. Quantitative approaches, such as representative surveys, emphasize coverage and the ability to generalize to larger populations. Triangulation, the combination of various methodologies in the study of the same phenomenon, is useful for validating results and for providing different insights into a selected subject area.

ACTION RESEARCH

There is a need for more action-oriented research that is integrally linked to social change. Research should have an action component that is identified by the subjects of the research themselves and is aimed at having an impact

International conferences will continue to be held year after year, while the lot of poor women and their communities remains bleak. It is not enough to assemble experts to lament these ills. It is important to act, to become alert, and to deliberate no longer. Change must happen at the local level where people make daily decisions that shape their lives and those of their children.

— Yianna Lambrou, International Development Research Centre, Ottawa, Canada (see Conway and Lambrou 1995)

on women's health status. It is not enough to simply ask questions and analyze problems in the traditional research style. Instead, researchers must "actively use their knowledge and skill to act and to bring about change in national policies and programmes" (Ellis 1986, p. 142). Indeed, according to Ellis (1986, p. 139), "any research done simply for its own sake and/or for the benefit of the researcher is oppressive and exploitative of those who are being researched."

State-of-the-art research data on women's health issues is often not integrated into public policy and health interventions. Atai-Okei (1994, pp. 205–206), for example, expressed frustration concerning the extent to which health research has failed to reach the local populations that it is meant to serve. Results from research are often not "put into practice in ... hospitals or in rural medical clinics."

Information obtained as a result of research must serve to empower women, and the communities to which the research applies, to foster the process of change (AbouZahr 1994, p. 6).

> All research on women's perceptions and needs in health should be designed and implemented with the express objective of developing interventions arising from the analysis of research results. Such interventions should be applied to extend health-care services into the community, improve the quality of health care available to women, and have an impact on women's health status.

Although there have been a number of health conferences, seminars, and workshops organized in the name of women's health in Uganda, little has been accomplished to date in terms of measurable improvement in the status of women's health or in the accessibility of health care to women.

— Hellen Rose Atai-Okei, Ateki Women Development Association, Kampala, Uganda

In addition to developing interventions, research results should inform public policies concerning health. However, many attempts by researchers to educate policymakers about the need to plan programs aimed at improving women's health and well-being "seem to have fallen on deaf ears" (Atai-Okei 1994). Violetta Lopez-Gonzaga (1995) has urged researchers to take that extra step and translate their "200-page documents that will just sit of the shelf for years" into "2-page documents that are useful to policymakers." Developing nations, she said, cannot afford to do research "just for the sake of it."

In her paper "WID, WAD, GAD," Rathgeber (1990b) states:

> The challenge of articulating the findings of ... research projects into viable, broad-based societal development plans and programs still remains to be met. To achieve this end, there is a particularly strong need for more effective communication and interaction among researchers, national and international policymakers, and donor agency representatives.

The results from two recent United Nations conferences represent major victories for women in the battle to ensure that women's concerns are integrated into policymaking. At the International Conference on Population and Development (September 1994, Cairo), women's groups from all over the world were successful in getting their message across that the population issue should be understood not as an isolated phenomenon, but in the larger framework of women's health and reproductive rights. Their success in placing women's concerns onto the international agenda resulted in a groundbreaking plan of action that stressed that if women are empowered to control their own reproductive lives, they will choose to have fewer children. In this regard, the plan of action stressed the importance of giving women equal participation in politics and public life and the need for initiatives to eliminate gender discrimination in the workplace as well as other forms of economic inequality, such as limits on a woman's ability to obtain credit, hold property, or receive an inheritance (UN 1994).

Likewise, despite intimidation and harassment from Chinese officials, women at the Fourth World Conference on Women (September 1995, Beijing) hammered out a 150-page Declaration and Platform for Action that built on the gains made at Cairo. In the weeks and months preceding the conference, activists were concerned that China's attempts to limit the participation of international nongovernmental delegates would set back important achievements made by women (Broadbent 1995). Indeed, as many as 10 000 women from NGOs who wished to participate in the conference were denied visas, and many others were prohibited from fully taking part. Despite the poor handling by China of the conference, women from around the world were able to turn the conference around.

> The program of action stemming from the ICPD [International
> Conference on Population and Development] stressed the
> importance of the advancement of gender equity, the
> empowerment of women, the elimination of all kinds of violence
> against women, and the importance of the ability of women to
> control their own fertility. The rights of women are an inalienable,
> integral, and indivisible part of universal human rights.
>
> — Trinidad S. Osteria, De La Salle University, Manila, Philippines

The final declaration forcefully denounced violence, domestic batter-
ing, and sexual harassment, and condemned rape as an instrument of war; it
upheld women's sexual and childbearing rights by denouncing forced sterilization, forced intimacy by spouses, and forced abortions; and it championed
women's economic empowerment by calling for women's access to financial
resources and banking credit. Women's health issues were linked to human
rights, and a broad approach to women's health was taken that emphasizes
social and gender determinants as well as a wide range of conditions that
negatively affect women's health (in addition to sexual and reproductive
health concerns). Furthermore, women from the governmental conference
and parallel NGO forum returned to their home countries committed to
making the declaration a reality.

WORKSHOP INITIATIVES

The workshops identified research gaps and produced recommendations for
further research in the area of gender, health, and sustainable development.
In addition, to help bring about changes in programs and policies related to
women's health, two action-oriented initiatives were developed.

Caribbean research agenda

At the workshop in the English-speaking Caribbean, a research agenda was
formulated to outline priorities for research on gender, health, and sustainable development. Recommendations for research addressed a number of priority issues including poverty, violence, nutrition and chronic diseases,
work-related health issues, and factors affecting the compliance and use of
services. Key policy issues were also outlined. These recommendations were
presented to the following key executing agencies: governments and their

ministries, the Caribbean Development Cooperation Committee, the Caribbean Community Secretariat, the Commonwealth Caribbean Medical Research Council, the Organization of Eastern Caribbean States Secretariat, the Pan American Health Organization and the World Health Organization, the International Development Research Centre, and the University of the West Indies.

The Asia and Pacific Women's Health Network

A highly ambitious action-oriented initiative was developed at the workshop in Singapore. A regional research and action network for women's health was launched. The objectives of the Asia and Pacific Women's Health Network are threefold:

+ To address fundamental gaps in knowledge about women's health at all stages of the life cycle;

+ To promote gender-sensitive health policies, research, and care delivery; and

+ To empower women in the articulation of their own health needs and their capacity to provide health care for themselves and for others.

At its most basic level, the network will serve as a clearinghouse for information on women's health and coordinate regional health research and activities that have a focus on women. At a more advanced level, the network will seek to bring together a critical mass of convergent effort on a comprehensive range of women's health issues to improve the health and well-being of women of the region. The network will give special attention to health issues that have resulted from the rapid economic development of the countries in the region. The network will bring together practitioners, policymakers, researchers, managers, and business interests in the region to address the fundamental gaps in knowledge about women's health issues, to access services at all levels, and to initiate innovative gender-sensitive programs.

A secretariat, based for the time being at ENGENDER,[3] will coordinate activities and disseminate information through these activities:

+ Information gathering and information sharing: building databases, coordinating and producing a network newsletter, showcasing success stories and lessons learned, and developing and managing an electronic bulletin board;

---

[3] ENGENDER is the Centre for Environment, Gender and Development, an NGO based in Singapore that jointly hosted the workshop with IDRC.

✦ Research: coordinating transnational research activities;

✦ Advocacy and coordination of strategies: coordinating advocacy of policymakers at the international, regional, and national levels;

✦ Training and education: developing training modules about gender sensitization and sharing training materials and modules that can be translated, popularized, and tailored to local needs; and

✦ Facilitation of funding.

Task forces were formed on several issues: occupational health; AIDS; osteoporosis; environmental health; health-care systems; tropical parasitic diseases; reproductive health; and women against tobacco. Furthermore, strategy-based task forces were also proposed on: women's empowerment and participation; sustainable mechanisms of development; community-based research; policy advocacy; and communications and information dissemination.

Chapter 4

AIDS

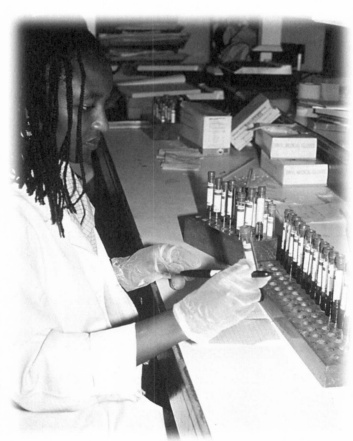

As we move forward through the second decade of AIDS infections, we must ask ourselves: "Have we really learned from this disease?"

— Arletty Pinel, GENOS International, São Paulo, Brazil

AIDS — acquired immune deficiency syndrome — is a major public health issue in most regions of the world. AIDS is a disease defined by a set of signs and symptoms, caused by HIV (human immunodeficiency virus), and characterized by a compromised immune response. HIV, which is transmitted through body fluids (semen and blood), produces a defect in the body's immune system by invading and then multiplying within white blood cells.

Since the identification of the HIV virus over 14 years ago, there has been a substantial growth in the number of people affected by this disease. An average of 6 000 people per day — over half of them women — are infected with HIV (World Bank 1993). The World Health Organization's Global Programme on AIDS estimates that more than 17 million people have been infected with HIV since the beginning of the pandemic. Of those, there are an estimated 4 million AIDS cases (WHO and UNDP 1994). The World Health Organization has predicted that by the year 2000 there could be as many as 26 million people affected by HIV and AIDS worldwide (World Bank 1993). However, it emphasizes that "given the short time it takes infection rates to double in many developing countries and the rapid spread of the disease to countries that previously had low numbers of infections," the total figure in 2000 may be two to three times higher than the above projection (World Bank 1993, p. 99).

Although the AIDS epidemic is a major concern in many regions of the world, some areas have been more profoundly affected than others (Figure 2). In 1990, more than 80% of those infected lived in developing countries, and this figure is expected to increase to about 95% by 2000 (World Bank 1993).

Sub-Saharan Africa has been hardest hit by the AIDS pandemic and accounts for over two-thirds of the total worldwide number of people infected with HIV. As of mid-1994, WHO estimated that over 10 million HIV infections had occurred in Africa. In certain cities in Africa, the prevalence of infections is as high as one in three. Northern Africa, however, is an area that currently has a relatively low level of HIV infection.

AIDS was not recognized as a serious health issue in Asia until the late 1980s. However, the progression of HIV infection is now faster in Asia than in other regions of the world. As of mid-1994, WHO estimated that there was

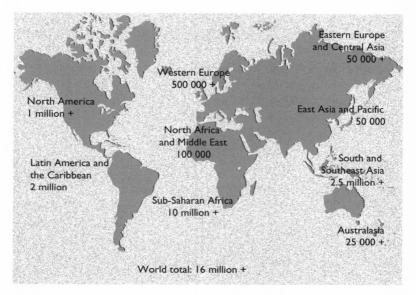

Figure 2. Estimated distribution of total adult HIV infections
(source: WHO and UNDP 1994).

a cumulative total of over 2.5 million HIV infections in this region. India and Thailand account for the majority of infections.

In Latin America and the Caribbean, 1.5–2 million people are believed to be infected. Brazil and Honduras are the worst affected. HIV infections in this region are largely concentrated in urban areas.

With regard to HIV and AIDS statistics, it is tremendously difficult to assess the true extent of the epidemic because of the high levels of under-reporting. For example, according to epidemiologists, the rate of under-notification in São Paulo, Brazil, may be as high as 100%, and the number of HIV positive people may be as many as five times the number of officially reported cases (Goldstein 1994).

INFECTION LEVELS AMONG WOMEN

Since 1981, the pattern of transmission of HIV has shifted considerably. In certain regions of the world, AIDS was originally thought to affect mainly homosexual males, prostitutes, and drug users who shared needles. Married women, or those with steady partners, were believed to be at a relatively low risk of HIV infection through sexual transmission.

In recent years, however, the number of women infected with HIV throughout the world has increased dramatically. In 1994, the number of women infected with HIV exceeded 6 million worldwide. The World Health Organization estimates that there are currently 115 000 HIV-infected women in North America, 425 000 in Latin America and the Caribbean, more than 4 million in Africa, and about 1.8 million in Asia and the Pacific (Figure 3). By 2000, it is expected that the number of infected women will equal that of men (Panos Institute 1990).

In North America and Europe, women have remained a relatively small percentage of the total number of HIV-infected people. However, the rate of infection among women is on the rise. In 1994, 18% of all AIDS cases in the United States were women (up from 7% in 1985) (Cohen 1995). The Centers for Disease Control in the United States said that cases among women are increasing by roughly 17% a year, and growing numbers are contracting AIDS through heterosexual contact (New York Times 1995, p. 11). In the United States, minority women are consistently affected more often. Blacks and Hispanics account for over 75% of reported cases among infected women (Campbell 1990; Carpenter et al. 1991).

In sub-Saharan Africa, more than one-half of newly infected adults are women, and over 1 in every 40 adult women is now infected. Between 60 and 80% of infected women are monogamous and have been infected by their

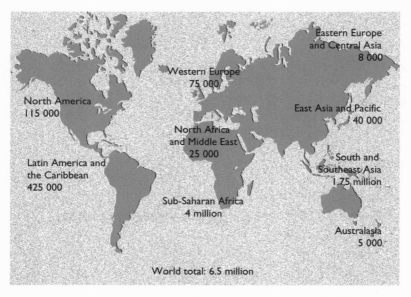

Figure 3. Projected distribution of HIV-infected women (excluding AIDS cases) in 1995 (source: WHO and UNDP 1994).

husbands (Hatcher Roberts and Law 1994). In Uganda, more than 60% of infected persons are women, and in Kampala, more than 30% of all pregnant women are infected (World Bank 1993). The HIV status among prostitutes in Kenya has reportedly risen from zero in 1980 to 88% in 1988 (Ngugi 1991, cited in Koblinsky, Timyan et al. 1993).

In Asia, as in Africa, almost half of all newly infected adults are women. The commercial sex industry in many Asian countries (such as Thailand and India) is closely related to the heterosexual transmission of HIV from female sex workers to male clients and vice versa.

In Latin America, initially, the most profoundly affected by AIDS were homosexual men, bisexual men, and injecting drug users. However, heterosexual contact now accounts for 75% of all new infections. One-quarter of all HIV infections are among women. In Brazil, the percentage of reported AIDS cases attributable to heterosexual transmission increased from 7.5% in 1987 to 26% in 1993–94. In Peru in 1987, the ratio of AIDS cases among men and women was approximately 15 to 1. In 1993, the male to female ratio was 7 to 1 (Chauvin 1993).

TRANSMISSION AND EFFECTS OF HIV AND AIDS

The main mode of transmission for AIDS in developing countries is through heterosexual intercourse, which accounts for more than 85% of infections (World Bank 1993). As well as through sexual intercourse, an individual can be exposed to HIV by contact with contaminated blood.[4] AIDS can also be transmitted from mother to child during the perinatal period. Approximately 30% of babies born to HIV-positive mothers are infected with the virus (WHO and UNDP 1994). Babies can also contract HIV through breast milk (World Bank 1993).

Casual transmission from person to person does not occur. AIDS is not transmitted by kissing, embracing, coughing or sneezing, or by sharing dishes or clothing. HIV may live in the human body for years before actual symptoms of AIDS appear. It takes 6–10 years, on average, for an HIV-infected adult to develop AIDS (World Bank 1993).

AIDS is a syndrome in which "the body's immunity goes berserk" (Usher 1992). AIDS weakens the natural defence system that usually regulates the body. It causes disease primarily by lowering the resistance of the body to fight other infections that can be fatal. The body eventually dies because,

---

[4] Such as from blood transfusions or through exposure to HIV-infected blood products, such as syringes and infected medical instruments.

> *For women, the chief mode of transmission of HIV is heterosexual contact.*
>
> — Anna Strebel, University of the Cape, Belleville, South Africa

vulnerable to the slightest infection, it can no longer protect itself. As described by Usher (1992, p. 26):

> People infected with the human immune deficiency virus fall prey to ailments that a normal healthy person might barely notice. People with AIDS die of tuberculosis, they die of cancers and pneumonia, they die of internal haemorrhaging, they die because wounds inflicted from a bump or a fall never heal but just get worse .... A person with AIDS can die from the common cold.

TREATMENT AND PREVENTION

There is no effective treatment, and no cure. Although numerous efforts are currently under way in the search for a cure, the prospects of success are far on the horizon. Studies are being done with antiviral drugs such as azidothymidine (AZT), but these drugs are prohibitively expensive for most people in developing countries.[5] Antiviral drugs also have severe side effects, and may, at best, slow down the progress of infection and marginally prolong life (do Prado 1994). Most treatment focuses on the alleviation of pain and the management of opportunistic infections that afflict HIV-infected persons, such as tuberculosis, diarrhoea, and candidiasis.

In the search for a cure, researchers must be cognizant that any vaccine must be appropriate for use in developing countries. A vaccine based on HIV strains commonly found in Europe and the United States would be of limited use in developing countries. Furthermore, an effective vaccine would have to be easy to distribute and affordable to all.

With no definitive cure or treatment for AIDS, prevention is the only way to fight the spread of HIV transmission. Currently, the main prevention methods are as follows:

✦ Providing information on how to avoid infection (such as reducing the number of sexual partners and modifying high-risk sexual behaviour);

[5] According to the World Bank (1993), 1 year of AZT costs more than US $3000.

✦ Promoting the use of the male latex condom, which is effective in preventing the transmission of HIV when it is used in a consistent and correct fashion;

✦ Treating other sexually transmitted diseases; and

✦ Reducing blood-borne transmission.

STDS AND HIV TRANSMISSION

With the recent worldwide focus on HIV and AIDS, other diseases that are transmitted primarily by sexual contact have received less attention. Sexually transmitted diseases (STDs) are extremely common infections. According to a 1990 estimate by WHO, there are more than 250 million new cases each year worldwide. An increased risk of acquiring an STD is related to the following factors: young age of first sexual intercourse (which increases the number of years of sexual activity and the probability of exposure to a number of partners), multiple partners, a relationship with a partner who has a history of multiple partners, and lack of appropriate protective contraception (RCNRT 1993).

The female reproductive tract appears to be particularly vulnerable to organisms transmitted during sexual intercourse. Male-to-female transmission of some STDs is at least 15% more efficient than female-to-male transmission (WHO and UNDP 1994).

STDs have severe and often irreversible consequences that disproportionately affect women. Untreated STDs in women can lead to pelvic inflammatory disease, infertility, increased risk of ectopic pregnancy, spontaneous abortions and stillbirth, premature delivery, and acute or chronic infections in infants born to infected mothers (RCNRT 1993).

The presence of STDs also greatly increases the probability of HIV transmission. Individuals with an STD are two to nine times more likely to become HIV-infected through intercourse with an infected partner, than those who do not have an STD (Population Reports 1990). In 1991, 54% of all STD patients at an STD clinic at Zambia's University Teaching Hospital and 60% of STD patients at an urban health centre in Kariba, Zimbabwe, tested positive for HIV. Nearly one-third of the patients in an STD clinic in Bombay, India, were HIV positive in 1991 (Panos Institute 1992).

HIV transmission is facilitated by the genital lesions and inflammation associated with STDs. The probability of HIV transmission is most pronounced with the presence of a genital ulcerative condition (Germain 1991; Bassett and Mhloyi 1993), although there is growing evidence that nonulcerative cases can also increase the probability of HIV transmission.

With regard to vaginal discharge, women often receive little or no information regarding its genesis, how it is transmitted, how it can be treated, or how it can be prevented. Most affected women are convinced that vaginal discharge is a natural part of being a woman, and that they are condemned to suffer from it for life, particularly if they maintain an active sexual life.

— Leda Pesce, Paulina Luisi Movement, Melo-Cerro Largo, Uruguay

Because of the role of STDs in AIDS transmission, many experts and international organizations have emphasized the importance of controlling STD infections (World Bank 1993; Lwihula 1994). However, the importance of STDs as cofactors for HIV transmission, especially for women, continues to be overlooked (Dixon-Mueller and Wasserheit 1991). From the perspective of the woman, chronic vaginal discharge is often seen as a "normal female complaint" related to her intimate life, one of the many "natural" discomforts associated with being a woman (Guimarães 1994; Pesce 1994; Vlassoff 1994).

STDs in women often go undetected and therefore untreated (Mhloyi and Mhloyi 1994; Ngwenya 1994). Sometimes physicians fail to distinguish an abnormal discharge from normal secretions. Although most STDs cause painful symptoms in men, women are more likely to harbour asymptomatic infections for prolonged periods — indeed, 50% of STD-infected women have no external symptoms whatsoever (Nowak 1995). This has serious consequences for the health and well-being of women and also results in an increased vulnerability to HIV infection (Standing and Kisekka 1989).

The current emphasis on AIDS should not let us marginalize or ignore other STDs. A sizable proportion of the population, particularly young girls and boys, still lack adequate information about STDs. Educational programs need to focus on the link between HIV infection and STDs and educate women and men, and young girls and boys, about how to prevent STDs,

The presence of sexually transmitted diseases has been shown to increase the risk of HIV infection. In women, symptoms of a STD are often less apparent than in men. STDs in women often go undetected, and therefore untreated, which results in an increased vulnerability to HIV infection.

— Anna Strebel, University of the Cape, Belleville, South Africa

recognize symptoms, and how and where to seek appropriate health care related to STDs. Restrictions that exist in some societies and prevent adolescents, particularly young women, from having access to information on sexuality, contraception, and disease prevention must be overcome (Pino et al. 1994).

THE AIDS EPIDEMIC AND WOMEN

The AIDS epidemic has had particularly harsh consequences for women in developing countries. Because women are usually the primary caretakers of family members, household illness often means that greater demands are placed on women (Wilson 1993). Women must care for infected family members and continue their already substantial duties in the home and in the formal employment sphere. Danziger (1994, p. 913) points out:

> As the number of people with AIDS within a given household rises, and growing numbers of orphans and other dependents are taken in, so the female head together with other women in the household are required to spend more and more time on care provision.

Women may also have to take up the activities of sick household members, which means that their working days become longer, their work loads heavier, and some of their own activities may have to be deferred (Durana 1994). "The enormous burden of care placed upon women by the AIDS epidemic ... will eventually force many women to neglect some of their other responsibilities, including their own health and well-being" (Danziger 1994, p. 913). Support and resources for those involved formally or informally in the care of sick and dying HIV-infected individuals are urgently required.

Many AIDS victims are heads of households, which has disastrous implications for families. In Uganda, for example, the highest incidence of AIDS cases occurs among adults between the ages of 16 and 42 (Wawer 1991), the most productive members of society. The illness of a wage earner in the household, who is often male, means that the household loses the person's labour, as well as the income deriving from their job (Adeokun 1994; Tsikata 1994).

When a woman develops a HIV-related illness, fulfilling her responsibilities becomes difficult or impossible. The implications for the family are particularly acute in cases where women are heads of their households and responsible for the day-to-day problems of securing support. Families that depend on women for the maintenance of subsistence crops, for example, often face a radical reduction in the availability of food within the household (Danziger 1994). In some cases, a woman's role on the farm may be replaced by the labour of older children, particularly girls, who are removed from school for this purpose.

When a household member develops AIDS, extended family members may interfere to the detriment of the woman. She may be accused of being the cause of the infection and treated in a cruel fashion by meddling relatives, even if she is not responsible for the illness. An HIV-positive women is often assumed to have had multiple partners or to have engaged in prostitution, and she is therefore considered a "bad woman" (WHO and UNDP 1994). She may be relocated to her parental home as a way of reducing her burden on the marital household and denied the custody of her children. The repercussions can be particularly devastating if her illness is, in fact, traceable to previous sex work (Agyeman 1992; Anarfi 1992).

HIV-positive women may suffer violence or abandonment often at the hands of their husbands (Danziger 1994). Hamblin and Reid (1991) reported that "[o]ften relatives will encourage a man who appears fit and well to leave his wife with AIDS and find another, with no understanding that he may pass the infection on to another woman."

In a few cases of HIV-positive women [in relationships with noninfected men], males have received direct pressure from their own families to abandon their partners.

— Rafael Garcia, Autonomous University of Santo Domingo, Dominican Republic

---

In areas of the world that have been worst affected by AIDS, the rapid sequence of deaths of adult household members has resulted in the total collapse of households. Tragically, high levels of orphanhood and child destitution have resulted (Adeokun 1994), and the older generation has been left with the burden of raising orphans. Gender inequality could result in the differential treatment of female and male orphans: "When caretakers can only afford to send a few children to school, female orphans will probably be disadvantaged; grandparents may also keep older girls at home to help even if funds are available" (De Bruyn 1992, p. 255).

Certain cultural traditions can further exacerbate the terrible effects of the AIDS epidemic. In some patriarchal societies, for example, when a husband dies, in addition to the emotional suffering created by the loss, women have no traditional rights of ownership to their husbands' property. This creates enormous hardship for surviving family members (Adeokun 1994).[6]

---

[6] See Manneschmidt, S., "AIDS programs in Uganda: what lessons can be learned for Nepali women?" Unpublished paper submitted to the 1994–95 TDR/IDRC competition.

Moreover, "even when inheritance laws upholds women's rights to their husband's property, customs which surround inheritance practices may be such that widows are coerced into conceding their inheritance to the families of their deceased husbands" (Danziger 1994, p. 913).

Appropriate policy initiatives are needed to change deleterious social and legal traditions [such as the] unfairness of inheritance systems. Governments need to move beyond the rhetoric of gender equality and make the necessary legal modifications to traditional practices that so patently deny equality to women.

— Lawrence A. Adeokun, Makerere University, Kampala, Uganda

THE TRANSMISSION OF AIDS AMONG WOMEN

Biological factors

There is increasing evidence that women are biologically more likely to acquire HIV infection through heterosexual intercourse than men (Mantell et al. 1988; Rodin and Ickovics 1990; UNDP 1992; Adeokun 1994). WHO and UNDP (1994) reported that studies in many countries have found that male to female transmission of HIV appears to be two to four times as efficient as female to male transmission.

There are a number of dimensions of the female reproductive system that make it more conducive than the male anatomy to HIV transmission: the concentration of HIV is greater in semen than in vaginal secretions; the vagina is more susceptible to infections than the penis; and, anatomically, with unprotected intercourse, women are the depositories of seminal fluids (do Prado 1994; Pesce 1994). The fact that prevalence of HIV infection is highest in women aged 15–25 years[7] has led to the suggestion that the intact but immature genital-tract surface in young women is less efficient as a barrier to HIV than the mature genital tract of older women (UNDP 1992). Furthermore, decreased mucous secretion among young and postmenopausal women provides less assistance in minimizing irritation and tearing of the

---

[7] In men, HIV infection peaks 5 to 10 years later in the 25–35 year age group.

genital membranes and can facilitate viral entry among these women (UNDP 1992; do Prado 1994; Pesce 1994; WHO and UNDP 1994). Sexually transmitted diseases and gynaecological infections also leave the female vulnerable to AIDS (do Prado 1994).

HIV does not seem to progress more rapidly in pregnant women than in nonpregnant women, at least in the early stages of infection (Strebel 1994). Pregnancy, in the absence of HIV-associated symptoms, does not strongly influence disease progression (Carpenter et al. 1991; Hankins and Handley 1992). However, because of their childbearing role (involving pregnancies, abortions, and births), women run a significant risk of receiving blood transfusions and other blood products that, without adequate blood-screening procedures, may be contaminated with HIV (Pesce 1994).

Women frequently have a poorer prognosis once infected and die sooner than men (Jones and Catalan 1989; Berer and Ray 1993). This may be related to the fact that the progression of AIDS is associated with the basic health and immune status of the individual prior to infection, and women tend to have poor general health and nutrition (Adeokun 1994). Inadequate nutrition not only slows the healing process and depresses the immune system, it can also inhibit the production of mucous (UNDP 1992).

It is difficult to discern whether the poor prognosis of women, compared with men, is related to biological differences or is connected to the fact that women tend to be diagnosed later than men and usually present for medical help later than men (Hankins and Handley 1992). A recent American study, which followed 768 women and 3 779 men over a 15-month period from 17 health centres around the United States, reported that women suffering from AIDS had shorter survival rates than men and were particularly susceptible to pneumonia, a main killer of infected victims. The researchers stated that the increased risk of AIDS-related pneumonia among women might have been associated with their relative lack of access to health care, their lower socioeconomic status, and their limited access to the social support available to infected men (Melnick et al. 1994).

Urgent research is needed to explore the possibility of a physiological basis to the susceptibility of infection in women. For example, research should examine whether the shorter period between diagnosis and death for women, in comparison with men, reflects factors such as delayed diagnosis in women, a lack of knowledge about the early symptoms of HIV infection in women, or more rapid progression of the disease (Paolisso and Leslie 1995).

Misconceptions about AIDS

Lack of complete information and understanding about AIDS

Many researchers have pointed out that although there appears to be a wide-spread general awareness about the basic messages surrounding AIDS, in many instances, there is a lack of detailed or thorough understanding about the disease (Adeokun 1994; Guimarães 1994; Mhloyi and Mhloyi 1994; Pinel 1994; Kuyyakonond 1995). Adeokun (1994) and Mhloyi and Mhloyi (1994) reported that, in their respective countries (Uganda and Zimbabwe), nearly 100% of people were aware of AIDS and understood the central role of the condom as a method of preventing the transmission of the virus. Mhloyi and Mhloyi reported that there were no marked sociocultural differences in AIDS awareness and that a basic comprehension could be found across all age, sex, and marital groups. However, both researchers found that, despite the fact that people had been bombarded with basic information, they continued to be ill-informed. For example, Mhloyi and Mhloyi found that approximately 36% of the respondents reported that they did not know the difference between HIV seropositivity and AIDS, and 32% reported that there was no difference. Only 13% said that a HIV positive person was healthier than one who was suffering from AIDS (Table 1).

Data from Mhloyi and Mhloyi's study also revealed that there were a number of misconceptions about the causes of AIDS. Only 19% of the respondents understood that AIDS was caused by HIV, and only 11% reported multiple sex partners as a determinant of HIV infection. Consistent with the frequent belief that sexually transmitted diseases are a "woman's disease" and that women are "reservoirs of infection" or "vectors of transmission," whereas men are victims, the majority of respondents thought that AIDS was caused by women, prostitutes, and soldiers (Table 2).

A survey in Tanzania revealed that 15% of respondents believed AIDS was an unpreventable punishment from God, 10–12% thought AIDS could be contracted by touching the body or wearing the clothes of a person who died

Table 1. Survey results: "What is the difference between someone who is HIV positive and someone who is suffering from AIDS?"

Response	Frequency (%)
Don't know the difference	35.9
There is no difference	32.1
HIV-positive victim is healthier	13.1
Not sure	3.4
HIV-positive victim can be cured	0.9
Other	2.1

Source: Mhloyi and Mhloyi (1994).

Table 2. Survey results: "What causes AIDS?"

Response	Frequency (%)
HIV	18.9
Women	21.4
Men	5.9
Prostitutes	16.8
Soldiers	11.6
Truck drivers	3.8
Many sexual partners	11.0
Other	10.5

Source: Mhloyi and Mhloyi (1994).

of AIDS, 25% believed AIDS could be transmitted through mosquitos and other insect bites, and 20% said the disease only affected prostitutes, barmaids, and long-distance truckers (Ndejembi 1993).

In Mhloyi and Mhloyi's study, there was a greater understanding of AIDS symptoms. Weight loss was identified as a symptom of AIDS by 53% of respondents, 38% recognized continuous illness, and 2% had no awareness of the symptoms of AIDS.

Some people may act on insufficient and incomplete information, much to their detriment. In the words of one 30-year-old man who purported to know a great deal about AIDS, "Since I got to understand more about AIDS, I only go out with younger girls, or even married women if I can; no more prostitutes" (Mhloyi and Mhloyi 1994, p. 18). Some men had a lack of comprehension concerning the latency period of HIV infection. They believed that "these days you have to be careful with the choice of partners" and said that they took precautions "by picking a woman you see is AIDS-free" (Mhloyi and Mhloyi 1994, pp. 13, 18).

A study of rural women in Northeast Thailand also found that women did not understand that there was a latency period between the time of infection and a positive HIV test. Some women felt that their husbands were safe

---

The results are consistent with the cultural belief that sexually transmitted diseases are a "woman's disease," and that women are vectors whereas men are victims. The association of AIDS with "high-risk" sexual groups is a belief that serves to distance HIV infection from the mainstream population.

— Gilford D. Mhloyi and Marvellous M. Mhloyi, University of Zimbabwe, Harare, Zimbabwe

because they had been tested before they returned home after an extended absence. Other women stated that they used condoms "for a period following a husband's engagement with prostitutes" (Kuyyakonond 1995, p. 65). In the same study, some women said that they knew that they or their husbands were free of infection because they had been tested at some time in the past, indicating that they did not appreciate that the results from an old blood test may no longer be valid.

> Women who used condoms with their husbands reported that they used them only for brief periods directly following visits by their husbands to prostitutes — "until the danger has passed." Discussions revealed that these women did not see the risk of HIV-transmission as something continuous, but rather as something short lived and restricted to specific periods — following a husband's visit to a prostitute, and when symptoms become "especially bad."
>
> — Thicumporn Kuyyakanond, Northeast Centre for AIDS Prevention and Care, Khon Kaen University, Thailand

A study conducted in the Dominican Republic found that some men, believing that the risk of AIDS was related to commercial sex workers, avoided sexual relations with them, or "use[d] condoms when they believe[d] they [were] dealing with street-women"; however, with other women, such as less professional barmaids, they were less cautious (Garcia et al. 1994). Morris et al. (1994) reported that condom use was significantly less consistent with regular (multivisit) commercial sex partners than with casual (single-visit) partners. These are perfect examples of the extent to which "a little knowledge can be a dangerous thing." Men and women clearly need better quality education to dispel the myths and lack of depth of understanding about AIDS.

The association of AIDS with "high risk" groups

The association of AIDS with "high risk" groups, reinforced by educational and media campaigns, has served to distance HIV infection from the mainstream population (Usher 1992). Originally, AIDS was thought to affect mainly homosexual males, prostitutes, and drug users who shared needles. Despite the fact that the pattern of AIDS transmission has shifted considerably, in many societies there continues to be the misperception that AIDS is a "gay plague" (Guimarães 1994), a "peste gay" (gay pest) (Pinel 1994), the "pink plague" (Chauvin 1993), or the long-awaited divine punishment (Pinel 1994) meant to eradicate drug addicts, prostitutes, and homosexuals. In Brazil, for example, the archetypal AIDS patient is considered to be the prosperous white, male homosexual, working in the world of fashion, enter-tainment, or the arts. Language reflects this perception: the word *aidético*, which is used to refer to a person living with AIDS, implies homosexual behaviour (Guimarães 1994). Tragically, many people, struggling daily to lead "normal" lives, do not identify with media campaigns directed to "deviant" or "high risk" groups, and believe that they are not at risk (Guimarães 1994; Pinel 1994).

When asked who was at risk for AIDS, women most frequently responded that prostitutes and men who have sex with prostitutes were at risk. It is notable that very few women identified the wives of these men as a group at risk.

— Thicumporn Kuyyakanond, Northeast Centre for AIDS Prevention and Care, Khon Kaen University, Thailand

---

Given the perception that AIDS is largely a male disease, women who are not prostitutes may not acknowledge that they are at risk of AIDS infec-tion. According to Guimarães (1994), women interviewed in her study in Brazil often believed that their main risk of AIDS came from exposure to HIV-infected blood or objects that have had contact with blood (such as dental drills and syringes). Guimarães argued that because of the undue focus on the "scapegoats" of AIDS, the gender dimensions of AIDS among "normal" people have been overlooked. She said that, if we seriously want to conquer the AIDS epidemic, we must work toward a fuller understanding of the gender relations of "normal" people, rather than just focusing on certain "deviant" groups.

"Not my man!": The inability of women to accept that partners may be unfaithful

One of the recurring and highly troubling issues raised by many researchers concerned the fact that, despite evidence to the contrary, married women, or those in steady relationships, often do not think of themselves at risk of HIV infection. Many women have trouble accepting that their husbands or part-ners could have intercourse outside of their steady relationships, and expose them to the risk of HIV (do Prado 1994; Guimarães 1994; Mhloyi and Mhloyi 1994; Pesce 1994). This inability to view partners as possible infectors greatly reduces the possibility of preventive steps being taken by women (Pesce 1994).

One 35-year-old woman from Zimbabwe reported that, "the AIDS problem is for the men who spend time with prostitutes, this is not our problem" (Mhloyi and Mhloyi 1994, p. 18). Similarly, in a study conducted in rural Northeast Thailand, 77% of women, when asked who was at risk from the disease, reported that men having sex with prostitutes were at risk. It is notable that very few women (14.8%) identified the wives of these men as a group at risk (Kuyyakonond 1995). In the same study in Thailand, women who said that their husbands "did not travel" felt that they were not at risk. It was generally believed that travelling away from home was a time when men frequented prostitutes.

In Pesce's research study (1994) of poor women in Uruguay and Argentina, almost all the women interviewed submitted to the nonadoption of safer sex. Most women tended to believe that it was other women, and not themselves, who were exposed to the risk of AIDS, and they were unable to link their husbands or partners to "the men who fool around." One of the common HIV prevention methods cited by women in a Brazilian study related to the subjective choice and evaluation of partners. One woman at a family planning clinic in Brazil, when questioned about the risk of AIDS from her steady partner, replied, "but I know him!" (Guimarães 1994). Meanwhile, female AIDS patients at the Gaffrée University Hospital stated how misled they had been by their partners, what little knowledge they had about their partner's sexual life outside the home, and how they felt betrayed (Guimãraes 1994).

Some women apparently assume that marriage, or the state of being in love, protects them from this deadly disease (Pesce 1994). Women need to be educated to understand that, despite love and marriage, many men have intercourse outside of their steady relationships, and may expose their partners to the risk of HIV (do Prado 1994).

Brazilian culture nourishes a romantic fantasy where two individuals meet, fall in love, and become immune to all dangers. Love is almighty, and both men and women are seen as incomplete beings without the complement of each other. Sex is validated through love where there is no room for an infected prince or princess or the need to interrupt spontaneity with the latex of a condom. After all, everything can be justified for love, even death.

— Arletty Pinel, GENOS International, São Paulo, Brazil

Economic factors

Poverty of women's lives

Depending on various socioeconomic factors, some women are more likely to be exposed to HIV infection than others. There is a growing recognition that class variables, as well as race variables, intersect with gender to compound the complexity of power relations (Ramazanoglu 1989; Stamp 1989). In the United States, almost half the people who have been diagnosed as having AIDS are African-Americans and Latinos from impoverished urban neighbourhoods, and poor minority women are consistently most affected by AIDS. "In the U.S. especially, AIDS is disproportionately a disease of the dispossessed, a disease of the socially condemned and denigrated, a disease of social outcasts and a disease of the poor" (Singer 1994, p. 944).

Likewise, in Brazil, a large number of young, poor women, classified as either black or mulatto and largely illiterate, have become infected through HIV-infected partners (Guimarães 1994). In Ontario, Canada, sexually active teenagers from low-income families are much less likely to use condoms than teens from households with higher family incomes (Canadian Institute for Child Health 1994). Generally, evidence over the last two decades "points to the fact that powerless and poor groups of people (no matter where in the globe they exist) are ... more susceptible to the ravages of HIV" (Kambon 1995).

Poor women are likely to have reduced access to educational opportunities and decreased exposure to health-related information. Poverty contributes to poor nutrition and susceptibility to infection. Poor nutrition, chronic stress, and prior disease may lead to a compromised immune system and increased susceptibility to AIDS (Singer 1994). Women living in poverty are also less likely to receive an early diagnosis of HIV infection, and they frequently have limited access to health care and adequate treatment (Strebel 1992; Guimarães 1994).

Strebel pointed out that women often lack power and social status in society and, therefore, access to economic resources. As a result of their differential positioning in society, women are usually poorer than men, and are often economically dependent on men (Campbell 1990; Ankrah 1991; Ulin

A higher degree of female autonomy may result in wives being able to refuse sex from husbands who are HIV-infected.

— Lawrence A. Adeokun, Makerere University, Kampala, Uganda

1992). This lack of economic independence affects their ability to demand safer sex. In contrast, women with economic independence are more likely to be able to control the events of their sexual and reproductive health. According to a recent WHO document, "It is not coincidental that the countries in which the virus is now spreading fastest heterosexually are generally those in which women's status is low. Wherever sex discrimination leaves women undereducated, unskilled, unable to gain title to land or other vital resources in their own names and low self-esteem, it also leaves them especially vulnerable to HIV infection" (WHO 1994a, p. 59).

Poor women, concerned with economic survival, may not change their behavioral patterns, despite messages to adopt safer sex. AIDS statistics do not directly impinge on their lives. "Statistically, and in her own subjective view of the world, she is more likely to die of hunger, of a poorly done abortion, or other health complications before dying of AIDS" (Goldstein 1994, p. 919).

Over the past 15 to 20 years, Brazil has been facing a social, economic, and political crisis. This has resulted in several deleterious consequences including high rates of inflation, critical unemployment, constant lay-offs, low salaries, poor health care, chronic endemic diseases, and rising urban violence. These are immediate survival issues that are usually considered more pressing than the remote risk of HIV infection.

— Carmen Dora Guimarães, Universidade Federal do Rio de Janeiro, Brazil

Living and employment patterns

Living and employment patterns, as the result of economic imperatives, may have an impact on HIV transmission rates. In Zimbabwe, for example, there is a dual economy that is characterized by urbanized industrial centres and expansive agricultural communities that are connected by a well-developed communication infrastructure (Mhloyi and Mhloyi 1994). Family members are often separated for economic reasons as men go to urban areas to find work while women remain in rural areas. Couples can therefore spend a large proportion of their sexually active and reproductive years away from each other. Away from their partners, men often take a second wife or a girlfriend, or seek the services of a prostitute. A vicious cycle arises when migrants return home, bringing infections with them (Jacobson 1992b).

There have also been high levels of female migration from some countries as women search for work. For example, there has been widespread migration of women from the Philippines to surrounding Asian countries, the Middle East, and North America, to work as domestic labourers. These women may experience domestic violence and sexual abuse, and therefore be exposed to STDs, including HIV (Osteria 1995).

Prostitution

Despite the risks, women continue to engage in multiple sexual relations, often for economic reasons (Adeokun 1994; Lwihula 1994; Strebel 1994). As a result of the subordinated position of women in society, and their limited access to economic resources, commercial sex is an important source of income for many women struggling to survive with limited resources (Standing and Kisekka 1989; Pauw 1993). According to WHO (1994a, p. 59), "in hard times, some [women] find it necessary to trade sex for money, food, or shelter." Poor women who are under pressure not to refuse client demands for unprotected sex may be less able to insist on the use of condoms, thus increasing the risks of HIV infection (Schoepf 1988; Larson 1990; Strebel 1994).

In Brazil, for example, with growing inflation and poverty, an increasing number of young women in large urban areas, as well as men, have been drawn into the commercial sex market in search of an alterative source of income (Guimarães 1994). The epidemic is expanding rapidly in parts of Asia (such as Thailand and India), especially in countries known for their history of prostitution and for being affected by the impacts of international sex tourism (Ford and Koetswanang 1991; Rana 1991; Seraprespamni 1991). Random HIV testing of prostitutes in Bombay showed an increase from next to zero in 1986 to more than 25% in 1990 (Basnet Dixit 1990). A recent study conducted with prostitutes on Bombay's Falkland Road found that about 50% of the tested women were HIV positive (Manneschmidt, see footnote 6).

Feeding children and keeping a roof over their heads is high on [women's] agenda; even if it means sleeping with a new partner, for whatever support he gives during the period of time he spends with her.

— Asha Kambon, Economic Commission for Latin America and the Caribbean, Port of Spain, Trinidad (see Kambon 1995)

Economically destitute women and single-parent mothers who have entire economic responsibility for the members of their household, and less household income than male-headed homes (Schoepf 1988; Ulin 1992), may turn to sex work or prostitution (Anarfi 1992). According to one commercial sex worker, "the reason why I do this is because I have two children, no husband, and what else is there for me to do? I don't enjoy it, but I got no alternative" (Bledsoe 1990).

It should also be remembered that at least 100 million children live and work in the streets of cities across the world. Young girls from various parts of Nepal, for example, are sold by their parents and brought to urban centres, such as Bombay, India, to work as prostitutes (Manneschmidt, see footnote 6). These children live in extreme poverty, suffer from malnutrition and poor health, are often victims of exploitation, violence, and sexual abuse, and are at great risk of HIV and other sexually transmitted diseases (Panos Institute 1994a).

A few caveats

Strebel (1994) noted that some writers have warned against taking a simplistic analysis of the link between economic factors and AIDS. The complexity of the interrelationship between economics and AIDS can be seen in a number of ways. To begin with, some studies have found that women of higher economic status, who may have affluent, mobile husbands who are likely to pay for sex, also are vulnerable to HIV-infection (Larson 1990; Gwede and McDermott 1992).

Although some women are in single-headed households as a result of male abandonment, an increasing number of women are deciding to stay single because they believe that this strengthens their economic situation (Ramphele and Boonzaier 1988; Stamp 1989). According to Strebel (1994), these women may be in a better position to insist on condom use.

Sociocultural factors

Extramarital sexual relations

There are a number of traditions, contexts, and situations that involve the interchange of sexual partners, and which may increase the risk of STD or HIV infection. In many cultures, it is generally acceptable, even expected, for men to have sexual partners outside of marriage. In Thailand, for example, extramarital sex by husbands is a key factor in the transmission of HIV to wives (Pramualratana 1995).

In a survey conducted in Tanzania, four out of five men believed that it was a sign of manhood for a man to have extramarital sex (Ndejembi

1993). According to Guimarães (1994), the husband or steady partner who has extramarital relations may reason that what he does away from home is his own business, as long as he fulfills his prescribed role as protector of the home and provider of family needs. A man's sexual activity with other women is often seen as an expression of his virility.

Us men, we take AIDS as a joke. We are more happy-go-lucky. This is a man's nature; male chauvinism. When a man sees a woman, he forgets about AIDS. No matter what problem arises, the man says: "I can bear it." Many men feel that if the solution is not to have several women, they would rather die of AIDS. If you are a man and get AIDS, people support you and say: "He is a macho," because he got the disease by doing men's thing — sex with women. I myself used to believe AIDS was a tale, until I got a positive HIV test.

— HIV-positive man from the Dominican Republic, reported by Rafael Garcia, Institute of Human Sexuality, Universidad Autónoma de Santo Domingo, Dominican Republic

---

It has been estimated that between 50 and 80% of all infected women in Africa have no partners other than their husbands (Hatcher Roberts and Law 1994). In formally polygynous societies, males can justify extramarital relations, explaining that they might evolve into additional marriages (Adeokun 1994; Mhloyi and Mhloyi 1994). In societies where polygynous marriage practices do not exist or are on the decline, extramarital liaisons on the part of men are not uncommon (Mhloyi and Mhloyi 1994). One survey has shown that 75% of Thai men have had sex with a prostitute (Economist 1994). Other surveys in Thailand have shown that about six million Thai men use prostitutes each week and that condom use in brothels is inconsistent (Pradubmook 1994).

The cultural practice of postpartum sexual abstinence may also lead to multiple sexual partnerships on the part of the male. In some societies, although sexual abstinence after the birth of a child is proscribed for females, male are allowed to "graze around" (Mhloyi and Mhloyi 1994). Social and religious taboos that discourage intercourse between husband and wife while the women is menstruating or breastfeeding may also encourage men to seek extramarital partners (Jacobson 1992b). As well, throughout sub-Saharan Africa, traditional healers promote the idea that men infected with STDs should have sex with virgins to cure themselves (Jacobson 1992b).

Socially sanctioned practices that are used by men to justify oppressive practices toward women need to receive urgent but sensitive attention (Ramphele and Boonzaier 1988; Stamp 1989; Strebel 1994). As Ankrah (1991, p. 972) argues:

> The unassailable facet of African culture, the customary and legal right of males to unlimited numbers of partners, according to his wishes, should now be questioned as a value, because the heterosexual pattern of transmission puts all African men who have multiple partner sexual encounters at risk of HIV. Where culture and tradition, including polygamy, no longer advance a people, they should be jettisoned.

Although in some societies it is socially sanctioned for men to have sexual relations outside of marriage, this is generally not the case for women. However, in many societies, traditional practices and rituals exist that call for women to have extramarital sexual contacts. In parts of sub-Saharan Africa, for example, following the death of a man, one of the deceased man's brothers may "inherit" his widow. Intrafamilial sex may be sanctioned if the husband fails to impregnate his wife. Furthermore, a customary practice concerning the "sexual cleansing of widows" requires a widow to have sexual intercourse with a stranger. This is traditionally done immediately after the death of the husband to fend off haunting spirits of the dead husband (Lwihula 1994). Other situations where extramarital sexual contacts are reported to occur include the birth of twins and at weddings, where the bride's paternal aunt might have intercourse with the groom before the bride does (Balmer 1994). In areas where STDs and AIDS are endemic, these traditional practices, involving extended sexual networks, carry the risk of STD or HIV transmission (Lwihula 1994). Many societies are now faced with the dilemma of balancing the demands of traditions with acceptance of medical advice and technologies recommended by STD- and AIDS-prevention programs.

The Uganda Women Lawyers Association has been working to restrict, through the formal legal system, the cultural practice of a widow marrying her husband's brother. At issue is the perpetual marginalization of women, their inability to own property, and their right to be the primary guardians of their children.

— Seble Dawit, Independent Consultant on International Human Rights Law, New York, NY, USA (see Dawit 1994)

The implications of male bisexual relations

Male bisexuality, which exists throughout the world, poses particular difficulties for the prevention and control of HIV transmission: "There are married men who do not identify themselves as homosexual ... or bisexuals, but who have a fling with a ... gay man and then infect their wives" (Thomson 1994, p. 26). "It's the bisexual community that poses a greater problem [than the homosexual community], partly because those men are in denial of being at risk, and in denial of having homosexual relations with other men" (C. Jones, quoted in Ortiz 1994, p. 2).

In much of Latin America, a distinction is made between activos, men who insert during anal intercourse, and pasivos, men who receive (Singer 1994). Activos, although they engage in bisexual behaviour, view themselves to be heterosexual, while pasivos are considered to be homosexual (Carrier 1989; Singer 1994). Goldstein (1994) reported that, in Brazil, a large proportion of men are sexually active with both men and women but define themselves publicly (including to their female partners) as exclusively heterosexual. As a result, women are unaware of, or do not acknowledge, the bisexual sexual practices of their male partners.

Guimarães (1994) explored the issue of male bisexuality in Brazil and its implications for HIV transmission in women. Official statistics since 1982 have indicated that male bisexuality is related to a significant percentage of all AIDS cases. As of January 1994, 32.7% (13 084) of the reported cases of AIDS in men were the result of homosexual transmission; whereas, bisexual transmission contributed to 16.9% (6 773) of reported cases (Guimarães 1994).

In the past few years, a rise in the prevalence of HIV transmission in "low-risk" women[8] led to epidemiological investigations. These inquiries revealed that many women unknowingly had bisexual partners who were HIV-infected (Guimarães 1994). Despite statistics that have existed since the onset of the epidemic, the implications of male bisexuality for women have been grossly ignored by AIDS medical specialists, AIDS researchers, as well as those responsible for AIDS interventions (Guimarães 1994).

In the study conducted by Guimarães, women who were interviewed rarely suspected or mentioned that their partners might engage in bisexual behaviour. Many women, believing that their men were "macho" and "macho" men only wanted women, reported that their risk of AIDS rested solely with their partners' involvement with other women.

---

[8] "Low-risk" women are those who are married women or those with steady partners, between 20 and 40 years of age.

> *Since 1982, official statistics [in Brazil] have indicated that male bisexuality accounts for [a significant percentage] of all reported AIDS cases. Why was the female dimension of male bisexual relations so grossly ignored by AIDS medical specialists?*
>
> — Carmen Dora Guimarães, Universidade Federal do Rio de Janeiro, Brazil

Early sexual activity and early marriage

Early sexual activity plays an important role in the transmission of STDs. In many countries, over half of all HIV infections to date have been among 15–24 year olds, with a female to male infection ratio of 2 to 1. Indeed, the prevalence of HIV infection is highest in young women aged 15–25 years, and peaks in men 5 to 10 years later in the 25–35 year age group (UNDP 1992). High rates of infection in young females may be a result of early entry into marriage and early sexual relations.

Adolescents tend to believe that they are immortal and invincible and this poses a challenge to HIV-prevention strategies (Gray and House 1989). Recent studies suggest a trend toward increased sexual experimentation, by more adolescents, at a younger age, with more sexual partners (Cochran and Peplau 1991; Pino et al. 1994), and without the benefit of effective or regular contraception (Lema and Kabeberi-Macharia 1992).

The fact that women become infected at a significantly younger age than men has sparked a growing interest in discovering the reasons for this discrepancy. In addition to the possibility of a physiological basis, circumstances and situations in which young women have sexual intercourse are also relevant. For example, nonconsensual or hurried intercourse may inhibit mucous production and the relaxation of the vaginal musculature, both of which would increase the likelihood of vaginal trauma (UNDP 1992). As well, women often have sex with older men, who are more likely to be infected because they have been sexually active for a longer time. An increasing number of girls and young women are being encouraged or coerced to engage in sexual activities, as men select ever-younger partners in an attempt to reduce their risk of HIV infection. "There have been anecdotal reports of 'sugar daddies' waiting outside schools to offer money in exchange for sex to schoolgirls who may welcome the case so as to be able to buy supplies and other essential items" (Danziger 1994, p. 913). "Some exchange sex for stylish clothes and accessories which neither their poor parents, low wages nor petty trade provide" (Schoepf 1993, p. 1402). Men are also seeking out younger women for marriage with a view to protecting themselves from infection (Danziger 1994).

There is a need for further research concerning the relationship between onset of sexual relations and the pattern of HIV transmission. Strategies aimed at delaying the entry of females into sexual activity are clearly important, as are measures that increase the ability of young girls to control the situations in which they are sexually active. Neither young women nor young men should be pressured into early marriages or early pregnancies.

Successful marriage bonds in African settings are cemented by the bearing and rearing of children. A childless couple is often shunned and ridiculed. More often than not, the woman is blamed for the failure to have children, and is assumed to be infertile.

— George K. Lwihula, Faculty of Medicine, Dar es Salaam, Tanzania

---

Cultural importance of children

After marriage, there is considerable pressure for women to have children in all societies (RCNRT 1993; Garcia et al. 1994). Condoms, the main way to prevent HIV transmission, also control fertility, which presents a particular difficulty for women of child-bearing age. As Kathryn Carovano (1991, p. 136) noted, "To provide women exclusively with HIV prevention methods that contradict most societies' fertility norms is to provide many women with no options at all."

The grandmothers believed that the more children one has, the more helping hands you will have. Women believed that "children are treasures," and if you have no children, people would remark that you are a "barren and useless woman."

— Daw Win May, Institute of Nursing, Yangon, Myanmar

The main avenue for social legitimization for women in many societies is their role as mothers. Motherhood can provide women with their only "personal project," their only source of identity, and their only personal "possession" (Bonino 1994). Given the fundamental role that motherhood plays for many women, women who are aware of their HIV-positive status may become pregnant (Lwihula 1994), and they may also see this as a way to retain partners (Garcia et al. 1994). Furthermore, women with HIV-positive partners may risk infection to try to conceive (Garcia et al. 1994). One woman's strong desire for a child, despite her HIV status, was reported by Hamblin and Reid (1991):

> I am still hoping to have a child .... I have been told that it is totally self-ish, that I have no right to inflict the potential for suffering on an as yet unborn child. Who says I have no right? If I am lucky enough to fall pregnant, my child will be loved and wanted. Will that be further reason for my rejection by society?

Finally, cultural practices in some African countries that restrict certain funeral rights to those who have a child may provide further understanding as to why some HIV-infected women try to become pregnant.

The "right" of husbands to sex and sexual violence

In some societies, men dominate all decision-making in the household, and their dominance may include the "right" to sexual intercourse. In some African cultures, for example, it may be nearly impossible for a woman to refuse sex from her husband, even if she suspects that he has engaged in promiscuous sexual behaviour and that there may be a serious risk of HIV transmission (Bledsoe 1990; Lwihula 1993). A wife's refusal of her husband's "conjugal right" can be a legitimate ground for divorce (Adeokun 1994). In Zimbabwe, because a groom must pay money for his wife upon marriage ("bride price"), the woman is made to feel like a piece of property and often believes that she must give him "his money's worth" in terms of her sexual and reproductive capacity.[9]

Power relations in African couples clearly favour men. Men dominate decision-making in the household and their dominance extends to conjugal relations. Men may demand sexual intercourse even if it is against the will of their partners.

— George K. Lwihula, Faculty of Medicine, Dar es Salaam, Tanzania

[9] See Mhunga, R., "AIDS and violence against women." Unpublished paper presented at a seminar on the impact of HIV and AIDS on development, held 1 December 1994 at the International Development Research Centre, Ottawa, ON, Canada.

> *No matter how much knowledge a woman has, it is nearly
> impossible to overcome cultural hurdles, such as the traditional
> "rights" of husbands to the persons of their spouses.*
>
> — Lawrence A. Adeokun, Makerere University, Kampala, Uganda

Women, as a result of the "[s]ocial construction of traditional sex roles, together with women's limited control over their lives," (Strebel 1993, p. 39) are also exposed to the potential threat of sexual violence and the associated risk of HIV infection. Women who are raped face the possibility of contracting STDs, including AIDS, from an infected assailant (Berer and Ray 1993). A rape crisis centre in Bangkok reported that 10% of its clients contracted STDs as a result of rape (World Bank 1993). Young girls may also be victims of incest and sexual abuse by respected elders (teachers, for example). Societies should develop and enforce laws against rape and other forms of sexual violence.

Mutilation of female genitals

The practice of female-genital mutilation, popularly known as female circumcision, is widespread in 27 African countries, 7 Middle-Eastern countries, parts of Malaysia, India, and Indonesia, and among some immigrant populations in Western countries. An estimated 85 million to 114 million women in the world today have experienced genital mutilation. If current trends continue, more than 2 million girls will be at risk of genital mutilation every year (World Bank 1993).

Female-genital mutilation poses a plethora of health risks to girls and women: hemorrhage, tetanus, infection, urine retention, shock, and occasionally death (World Bank 1993). Possible transmission of HIV and other viral infections may occur when unsterilized instruments are used. For example, in rural areas, crude instruments such as dull knives, rusty razor blades, or shards of unwashed glass may be used (Omer Haski and Silver 1994). Moreover, infibulated women may be at greater risks of contracting STDs because tears are more likely during vaginal intercourse, and partners may practice anal sex if vaginal intercourse is impossible (De Bruyn 1992; van der Kwaak 1992). Because of the severe consequences that female-genital mutilation pose to women's health, women's groups in Africa have been working to end the practice (World Bank 1993). Other ritual practices, such as scarification, tattooing, and blood letting may also lead to HIV infection if performed with unsterilized equipment (WHO and UNDP 1994).

Vaginal drying

Vaginal drying or "dry sex" is a cultural practice that may contribute to significantly higher risks of infection among the women involved. To have "dry sex," women insert into their vaginas a variety of different agents (powders, herbs, cloth, aluminum hydroxide, rock salt, or stones) that are designed to tighten the vagina and dry up its natural secretions before sexual intercourse. Dry sex is based on the idea that the woman's vagina should be dry, tight, and hot to enhance sexual pleasure (Panos Institute 1994b).

The use of vaginal drying methods has been reported in Cameroon, Costa Rica, the Dominican Republic, Ghana, Haiti, Kenya, Malawi, Saudi Arabia, Zaire, Zambia, and Zimbabwe (Panos Institute 1994b). In rural areas of Zimbabwe, young women may be informed about dry sex by an aunt who is acting as a traditional educator at puberty or before marriage.

Dry sex probably increases the risk of contracting HIV during intercourse. The agents that are inserted into the vagina may cause irritation and damage. Increased friction augments the risk of genital ulcerations to both partners. Because condoms require some lubrication, and because they are likely to tear with excessive friction, the practice of dry sex makes it nearly impossible to use condoms (Panos Institute 1994b). More research about this sexual practice is urgently needed.

Unequal power relations between men and women

The subordination of women affects their decision-making in all areas of life, including sexuality (Pesce 1994), and plays an important role in HIV transmission. Gendered power relations influence the ability of women to take health-enhancing knowledge and translate it into preventive action. Men and women occupy different positions in society, and masculine and feminine gender roles are sharply differentiated. According to gender-role expectations, men should be active and dominant in sexual relations; whereas, women should take the passive and subordinate role. Women are socialized to believe that the "ideal woman" suppresses her desires to please her partner

Many women do not control how, when, with whom, and how often they have sexual intercourse. Women are socialized to believe that the "ideal woman" suppresses her desires and needs to please her partner.

— Elsa do Prado, Centro de Salud and Sexualidad "Alternatives," Montevideo, Uruguay (do Prado 1994), that her body is an object meant to satisfy men (Pesce 1994), and that she is valued for her sexually passive role. Many women do not control how, when, with whom, and how often they have sexual intercourse, but instead must submit to the judgements, opinions, decisions, and feelings of men (do Prado 1994).

To avoid infection, women are advised to abstain from sex, practice monogamy, or negotiate the use of condoms with their male partners. However, many women have a limited ability to influence the sexual activity of their spouses or partners (Strebel 1994). According to one woman from Zimbabwe, "what can we do, men will always graze around" (Mhloyi and Mhloyi 1994, p. 18). Women are asked to exert control and make choices in a domain where they have little control and few options (Hollis 1992; Strebel 1994).

These issues emerged in a study conducted in Cape Town, South Africa (Strebel 1994). Focus-group discussions were held with almost 100 black women (and a few men) from antenatal and STD clinics and community political organizations, and with domestic workers, teachers, and students. Gender issues were a dominant theme, particularly notions of power and responsibility. Many women stated that men had the power to determine the nature of sexual relationships. This meant that men had multiple sexual partners and women were not entitled to protest or to expect men to admit to this behaviour. It was recognized, however, that women did have some power and might also have multiple partners. Some women said that women could be more assertive and challenging regarding safer sexual practices. However, women saw many obstacles to challenging entrenched gender positions (Strebel 1994). Practicing safer sex was not an easy task because men largely did not take responsibility for prevention in the same way that they did not take responsibility for contraception. Because women generally took control of health issues, it was emphasized that a woman-controlled HIV-prevention method, which does not require male partner awareness, compliance, or action, was essential.

Difficulty negotiating condom use

Numerous researchers have addressed the various barriers that prevent the usage of condoms (Adeokun 1994; do Prado 1994; Garcia et al. 1994; Guimarães 1994; Lwihula 1994; Mhloyi and Mhloyi 1994). The inequality of power between men and women makes it difficult for women to suggest the use of condoms (Garcia et al. 1994; Guimarães 1994). According to Maria De Bruyn (1993), "prevailing power dynamics make self-protection by women problematic at best and very difficult or impossible at worst." AIDS-education programs need to acknowledge and find strategies to deal with the fact that women invariably have little or no say in sexual relationships and yet they suffer more severe consequences from reproductive health infections than men do (Germain 1991). Prevention strategies will continue to fail unless programs deal directly with these realities.

First and foremost, women and men need to be able to communicate effectively with one another. Most prevention and control measure require understanding and cooperation from both parties. However, there is often minimal or complete lack of communication between partners on everyday subjects, and there is even less dialogue on matters related to HIV prevention (Lwihula 1994). Furthermore, in many societies, there may be cultural restrictions preventing the discussion of issues surrounding sexuality (Ngwenya 1994; Manneschmidt, see footnote 6). In a study conducted in Thailand, little talk of condom use was reported among married couples, and half of the women said they would be embarrassed to ask for condoms (Kuyyakonond 1995). What talk did occur appeared to have been very limited and perfunctory. For example, women reported that their husbands had told them not to worry about AIDS because they had used condoms when they "went out."

Serious discussions about condom use within the marital relationship were rarely undertaken — wives rarely directly confronted their husbands about condom use .... Campaigns are needed to motivate married couples ... to discuss extramarital sex, to discuss perceived risks in contracting STD/HIV, and to discuss the need for condom use. Campaigns must promote such open discussions among married couples and emphasize that the initiation of such topics be undertaken by husbands, as a demonstration of their responsibility to their family.

— Anthony Pramualratana, Mahidol University, Nakornpathom, Thailand
(see Pramualratana 1995)

In a study of poor women from Uruguay and Argentina, Pesce (1994) reported that almost three-quarters of the women interviewed had talked to their partners about AIDS. However, because almost all of these women engaged in unprotected sex, Pesce suggested that the conversations were not very effective in encouraging the use of prevention measures. This raises the question of what exactly takes place when couples talk about AIDS. A greater understanding of communication patterns between women and men with regard to HIV transmission, as well as strategies to encourage more effective communication between partners, are essential. The lack of dialogue between partners on sexual matters suggests that there is an immediate need for interventions that bring women and men together to work on creating greater understanding of other points of view, reducing communication barriers, and initiating and sustaining behaviour change (Balmer 1994).

To be effective as an AIDS-prevention measure, condoms must be used correctly and consistency. However, men continue to resist condoms. As one women in a study by Mhloyi and Mhloyi (1994, p. 18) remarked: "If you want to get divorced, try asking your husband to use a condom."

Sometimes I want him to use it [a condom]. But he says why should he use it, he does not like that, and then he gets angry. Sometimes we quarrel. To even mention that he may get AIDS, he gets angry.

— A woman from Northeast Thailand, reported by Anthony Pramualratana, Mahidol University, Nakornpathom, Thailand (see Pramualratana 1995)

Condoms may be unacceptable to men for a variety of reasons. To begin with, condoms interfere with reproduction, and children are very important to both women and men in most cultures (Adeokun 1994; Lwihula 1994). In some sub-Saharan African countries, the average man wants to have more than 10 children, in part because large families serve as cultural symbols of a man's virility and wealth (Sachs 1994). Men also resist condoms because they are concerned about reduced sensitivity, and because they fear that using it will permanently interfere with fertility (WHO and UNDP 1994). Family-planning workers commonly report that suggestions of condom use are greeted with sayings such as "you can't wash your feet with your socks on," or "that would be like eating a sweet with the wrapper still on it" (Sachs 1994, p. 16). Also, because family-planning units tend to be women-oriented and accessible only to women, some men are reportedly upset when their wives bring home condoms because they have not participated in the decision-making process (Lwihula 1994).

Women encounter numerous difficulties when they attempt to introduce safer sex practices (Balmer 1994; do Prado 1994; Garcia et al. 1994; Guimarães 1994). Use of a condom clearly depends on the cooperation of the man because he is the one who "wears the condom." In many cultures, women depend on men to provide condoms because it may be socially inappropriate for a woman to carry condoms (Sacco et al. 1993; Garcia et al. 1994), and women may be reluctant to buy, carry, or keep condoms at home (Garcia et al. 1994).

> When a woman requests the use of a condom from a man, she
> is acting in a sexually assertive fashion, particularly if she
> provides the condom. This runs contrary to the role of the
> "proper" woman who is traditionally subordinate and passive,
> particularly in sexual matters.
>
> — Carmen Dora Guimarães, Universidade Federal do Rio de Janeiro, Brazil

To justify their request for condom usage, a woman may explain that the condom is necessary for contraceptive purposes. However, if a woman is married or in a stable relationship, she has other contraceptive options that can be used with no discomfort to her partner, such as the oral contraceptive, the intrauterine device (IUD), or sterilization. A woman may have difficulty justifying condom usage for anal sex because contraception is obviously not a consideration for this practice.

Although a woman can also explain that a condom is necessary to protect against STD (or HIV) transmission, this poses a challenge to the concepts of romantic love and fidelity (Strebel 1994), particularly if the woman is married or in a steady relationship. Permanent relationships usually operate on the assumption of monogamy, fidelity, and mutual trust. Suggesting the use of a condom, the "unwelcome symbol of extra-marital sexual activity" (Byron 1991, p. 29), implies that she suspects that her partner has been unfaithful. If her partner agrees to use a condom, her suspicion of infidelity is confirmed. A woman's suggestion to use a condom may also lead her partner to suspect that she has been disloyal, which may provoke a strong reaction from her partner, possibly involving physical punishment or desertion (Garcia et al. 1994; Guimarães 1994; Strebel 1994). According to a woman from Buwunga, Uganda, "If you advise your husband to use a condom, he may beat you and send you away. Where will you go then?" (Perlez 1990, p. A4).

Condom usage is also an issue for single women without regular partners. If a single women requests the use of a condom, her partner may believe

> Given their lack of power in gender relations, there is the
> danger that women who refuse sex or insist on condom use or
> fewer partners may face domestic violence.
>
> — Anna Strebel, University of the Cape, Belleville, South Africa

> *Condoms are distributed when they are available; unfortunately,*
> *the condom supply is often out of stock.*
>
> — Shirley Ngwenya, Health Services Development Unit, Acornhoek, North
> Eastern Transvaal, South Africa

that she is promiscuous or has a sexually transmitted disease, which may prevent the relationship from continuing. As one woman explained, "a good man is hard to find these days" (Guimarães 1994, p. 29). Single women, therefore, may be willing to take a chance by not using condoms and hope that love or luck will protect them against infection.

One highly disturbing fact is that condoms, the most commonly suggested prevention method, appear to be widely unavailable, particularly in remote areas (Lwihula 1994). Researchers from Africa, Asia, and Latin America have noted that limited family-planning services, lack of condom availability, or the high cost of condoms may make it impossible for those who wish to take preventive measures to do so (Adeokun 1994; Mhloyi and Mhloyi 1994; Ngwenya 1994; WHO 1995) This resource problem, which may be related to poor management and distribution, must be properly addressed.

> *Condoms appear to be widely unavailable. Many people*
> *reported a desire to use condoms, understanding their efficacy*
> *in reducing the chances of contracting a STD; [however], the*
> *majority of people often do not have access to condoms.*
>
> — Gilford D. Mhloyi and Marvellous M. Mhloyi, University of Zimbabwe,
> Harare, Zimbabwe

Fatalism and the irrational nature of love and sex

Individuals living in communities where AIDS is widespread can become complacent and fatalistic about AIDS. As people observe more and more people dying of AIDS, some may assume that they are also infected and decide that there is no use in altering sexual behaviour. According to individuals from Zimbabwe, "Death is with us, we can't run away from it" and "Well, we are all HIV positive, no one will remain, it is just a question of time" (Mhloyi and Mhloyi 1994, p. 18).

Finally, it must be remembered that people do not always deal with matters of sex and love in a rational fashion, and this may dramatically affect HIV transmission. AIDS interventions, however, have been devised based on the supposition that people will act in a logical manner if they are just given the right information. In the words of Keeling (1993, p. 307): "Our benign and hopeful assumption that reasonable people given reasonable information in a reasonable way would be reasonably likely to make reasonable changes in their behaviour to reasonably reduce their risks of acquiring HIV turned out to be unreasonable."

Individuals often take excessive risks when it comes to love and sex. Even when a woman is aware that her partner is HIV-infected, for example, she may not protect herself as a demonstration of her total, symbiotic link with her partner.

The pathology-centred rational approach to sexuality will never be enough to promote the understanding of the behavioural aspects in the spread of AIDS.

— Arletty Pinel, GENOS International, São Paulo, Brazil

INTERVENTIONS

Health education

Health education and prevention programs have been one of the main strategies used worldwide in the attempt to prevent the spread of STDs, including AIDS, and to increase awareness and understanding of these diseases. Initially, most programs focused on "high-risk groups," such as homosexual men, prostitutes, drug users, and truck drivers (Sekimpi 1988; Balmer 1994). In recent years, however, programs to spread information and change behaviour patterns have been increasingly directed to general populations, particularly young people who are starting to be sexually active (Balmer 1994; Manneschmidt, see footnote 6). The particular concerns of women have also started to receive more attention and service providers are currently struggling to develop and deliver gender-appropriate programs (Panos Institute 1990; Pearlberg 1991; Guimarães 1994).

Prevention programs aim to distribute information on how the virus is spread, and to inform people about the steps they can take to protect

It is inadequate to use counselling simply as an educational medium. Although counselling has had some success in educating individuals about the risks of STDs and AIDS, there needs to be more focus on the role of counselling to achieve sustained behavioural change.

— Don H. Balmer, University of Nairobi, Nairobi, Kenya

themselves against HIV infection.[10] These programs are based on the hope that education will lead to changes in behaviour patterns, and therefore to a reduction in STD transmission (Balmer 1994; Manneschmidt, see footnote 6).

Attempts to controls sexual behaviour through education, however, have not always proven successful. Even with correct, properly understood information, people may not change their actions. In a study of male truck drivers in East Africa with a 25% prevalence of HIV, 90% had sufficient knowledge of STDs and HIV, including knowledge of condoms and lower-risk behaviours (Bwayo 1991). Despite this knowledge, two-thirds of the men continued to engage in risky sexual practices.

Programs designed to increase adolescents' knowledge about HIV have also not eliminated high-risk behaviour (Baldwin et al. 1990). Available evidence suggests that adolescents continue to engage in high-risk sexual behaviour, even after participating in education programs (Thurman and Franklin 1990; DiClemente et al. 1992). Programs that attempt to promote the use of condoms as a preventive measure have only increased awareness, not usage (Jay et al. 1988).

Despite 14 years of the epidemic, most of the preventive actions are still limited to isolated projects that repeat the same elementary information. The federal government continues to rely on sporadic mass media campaigns, but their inconsistency, together with the dearth of complementary local interventions, has instilled the idea that AIDS is only a problem when there is an ongoing campaign.

— Arletty Pinel, GENOS International, São Paulo, Brazil

---

[10] For example, monogamy or reducing the number of sexual partners, choosing partners of lowest risk, avoiding contact with contaminated blood, using condoms, refraining from risky sexual practices such as anal sex, and treating STDs.

Media strategies

Although health beliefs can be influenced by media messages, the use of media to transmit complex information may be of limited effectiveness. Knowledge gained through the mass media is often incomplete, and it is of limited value because people do not have the opportunity to ask questions (Mhloyi and Mhloyi 1994). First-hand experience often has better success in promoting behaviour change (Mhloyi and Mhloyi 1994; Pesce 1994). Furthermore, many women may not benefit from information gained through educational campaigns in the media because the language used is not tailored to their level of education or cultural background (Pesce 1994). If media strategies hope to reach women, messages need to be appropriately targeted and tailored to the particular characteristics of women.

Poorly thought out media messages can create false impressions and be counterproductive. For example, many women do not believe that their partners could be possible infectors. This misperception can be reinforced by unclear media messages that promote monogamy as a way to prevent AIDS, and thereby lead some women to think they are not at risk of HIV transmission because they are only having sexual intercourse with one person. Health promoters need to exercise caution with these types of messages (Pesce 1994).

Some media methods may be better than others. Mhloyi and Mhloyi (1994) reported that exposure to radio was more likely to reduce the likelihood of STD infection than exposure to newspapers. Kuyyakonand (1995) also reported that women whose primary source of information was the radio tended to have more accurate information. This may be because live radio presentations, which often include question-and-answer sessions, may be more realistic to listeners (Mhloyi and Mhloyi 1994). Also, because of low levels of literacy, some women may not benefit from newspapers.

Public education programs need to identify channels of communication beyond the mass media to reach rural people. Many are too poor to buy a local newspaper, let alone a radio. Women tend to be more disadvantaged because they have little time to listen to the radio or read newspapers. Even if they had the time, many women are unable to read.

— Hellen Rose Atai-Okei, Ateki Women Development Association, Kampala, Uganda

Creative educational approaches

Given the lack of success of traditional educational campaigns, creative educational approaches are needed and information needs to be packaged in ways that make it interesting and relevant (Garcia et al. 1994; Manneschmidt, see footnote 6). More and more countries are using entertainment media, including soap operas, radio shows, and songs to encourage AIDS awareness (Heise 1993). Mhloyi and Mhloyi's study (1994), for example, experimented with different educational approaches including drama, the use of role models, songs, and discussions. These types of innovative approaches reduced communication barriers and informed people about key issues. The plays and songs were filled with conversation-provoking lines. For example, one line from the play read, "Theresa, don't you know that when you are in the middle of that business, you can barely think of a condom?" which encouraged the group to discuss obstacles to condom usage (Mhloyi and Mhloyi 1994). According to Asha Kambon (1995):

> New techniques need to be given greater prominence .... Popular theatre,
> [for example], can empower as it imparts new information and ... by its
> very meaning must be rooted in the culture of the people.

To educate and change risky behaviour in northeastern Thailand, IDRC-supported researchers, Thicumporn Kuyyakanond and Eleanor Maticka-Tyndale, pioneered an AIDS-awareness program that involved regular radio dramas on the subject of AIDS (Conway 1995). The radio scripts were based on stories taken directly from focus-group discussions and reflected real-life situations. The dramas, a mixture of soap opera and improvisational theatre, were styled after a traditional form of Thai theatre called Maw Lum. The project generated much interest and enthusiasm, and Thai health officials, in collaboration with local NGOs, expanded the pilot project to province-wide programs.

Our study experimented with different educational approaches including drama, songs, and discussions. We brought both men and women together from all age groups. These types of innovative approaches served to reduce communication barriers, as well as to inform people about key issues.

— Gilford D. Mhloyi and Marvellous M. Mhloyi, University of Zimbabwe, Harare, Zimbabwe

*Messages geared to women should focus on assertiveness
training and empowering women to protect their health.*

— Rafael Garcia, Universidad Autónoma de Santo Domingo,
Dominican Republic

Empowering women

Gender-power dynamics limit women's ability to determine the conditions under which sexual intercourse occurs. Many researchers have emphasized that the solution to AIDS "involves something much more profound than instruction in the use of condoms" (Usher 1992, p. 17), and one of the most important strategies to deal with AIDS is to increase the power and autonomy of women. Women need to be educated about their subordinate position in society, and encouraged to care for themselves: "The notions of self-care, and control over one's life, need to be felt at every emotional level, and not just rationally or intellectually imposed" (Pinel 1994, p. 57). As Usher (1992, p. 46) observes:

> Women in the age of AIDS, especially young women, must know her body well and understand her sexuality before she can be expected to discuss it with her future partner. AIDS requires women to make conscious, active decisions about the most intimate areas of their lives.

The difficulties encountered by women when they demand safer sex need to be explored with women , and strategies must be developed. Women need to be trained in how to use condoms and how to include them in sexual foreplay (Pesce 1994). It is also crucial that false beliefs be corrected through awareness-raising, such as the widespread misperception that husbands and partners are not infectors. At the Paulina Lousi Movement training program in Uruguay, for example, when women asserted that "men play around," program leaders probed this statement by asking "which men play around" to encourage women to consider the personal risk they may be exposed to (Pesce 1994).

Group counselling and training can be an effective format for helping women to deal with these issues. In a group, women are able to share common experiences and perceptions, examine values, gain support and validation for each other, and practice new behaviour skills in a safe environment (Moore 1981; Burden and Gottlieb 1987). Group training has been shown to improve the self-esteem of women, and may lead to a sense of empowerment (Weitz 1982). Jacobson (1992b) reported that several countries are now trying to bring women together to discuss taboos that may be harmful to

> Group counselling provides an effective format for helping women deal with self-concept issues. In a group, women are able to share common experiences and perceptions. Groups decrease isolation and provide a context where women can gain support and validation from each other.
>
> — Don H. Balmer, University of Nairobi, Nairobi, Kenya

their health. This empowers women because it breaks their silence and enables them to focus on the what is in their own best interest.

Throughout the world, women have always found strength in informal organizations, mobilizing themselves around specific activities, using kinship ties, neighbourhood groups, and other informal networks to accomplish their aims (March and Taqqu 1982; Ulin 1992). AIDS-prevention programs need to make the most of women's capacity for collective action. Heise and Elias (1995) argued that women who organize for change can help build group consensus and create a unified sense of purpose and possibility. In community organization projects, women can learn to analyze their situation and seek individual and collective solutions to their problems.

Female-controlled prevention measures

Given the incredible difficulty that women face in convincing men to use condoms, research is increasingly focusing on developing HIV-prevention methods that women can control. The recently available female condom, a polyurethane sheet with two rubber rings that secure it inside the vagina, still requires partner cooperation, and many women find it bulky and awkward to use (Panos Institute 1994b; Cohen 1995).

Although the spermicide nonoxynol-9 has been known to kill HIV in the laboratory for many years, there has been limited research on its protective effect against the sexual transmission of HIV. The first large-scale trial on

> Future research needs to explore prevention methods that women can control so they can protect their own health, as well as the health of their children.
>
> — Elsa do Prado, Centro de Salud and Sexualidad "Alternatives," Montevideo, Uruguay

American women is just beginning, and it will be several years before results are available.

The possibility of developing a virucide, a vaginally inserted microbicide that would protect against HIV transmission, while letting sperm pass unharmed, is currently being investigated. Such a product would allow women to protect themselves from HIV without their partner's knowledge or cooperation. However, this research is still in its very early stages (Panos Institute 1994b).

Interventions targeted to men

Most gender-based programs to prevent HIV transmission have focused exclusively on women. Although many AIDS interventions have targeted homosexual men, there has been limited attention placed on heterosexual men (Strebel 1994). However, because men have so much decision-making power in all areas of life, including sexuality, men need to be encouraged to take the initiative for prevention and be taught the importance of consistent and correct use of condoms.

> The exclusive focus on women in gender issues is not always in the interests of either women or gender equality. This has been clearly demonstrated in approaches to AIDS prevention for women. Male sexuality and power need to come under the spotlight if our analysis is to reflect the complexity of positioning in gendered power relations and AIDS-related behaviour. Without this, the solutions generated will involve unrealistic and unachievable options for the vast majority of women.
>
> — Anna Strebel, University of the Cape, Belleville, South Africa

In this regard, a recent study in Lima, Peru, suggested it may be important to use males as workers in the distribution of contraceptives, including condoms, to effectively reach men (Foreit et al. 1992). With the use of men in a community-based distribution program, the sales of condoms increased dramatically, as did the number of new male clients. Male distributers may have been particularly successful when working with male clients because they shared common characteristics with the population they served.

Likewise, the National Family Planning Council of Zimbabwe reported success with a 1989 intensive media campaign designed specifically to increase men's responsibility in family planning and to encourage joint decision-making among couples. The campaign included a series of informational and motivational talks by male educators. In addition, an entertaining serial drama about the consequences of irresponsible sexual behaviour was broadcast over the radio twice a week for 6 months and reached 40% of the male population in the country. At the end of the campaign, 40% of the men said that family-planning decisions ought to be made jointly by husband and wife, and 17% of the men who had attended at least one talk reported that they had started using a family-planning method (Sachs 1994).

> *Men should understand their own and women's reproductive health needs, share reproductive decision-making, and take more responsibility for reproductive health, contraceptive use, and their families' welfare.*
>
> — Trinidad S. Osteria, De La Salle University, Manila, Philippines

Early and complete treatment of STDs

Promotion of the early and complete treatment of STDs is one of the key strategies to prevent HIV transmission. However, many STD-control programs have had little success (O'Connor et al. 1992; Lwihula 1994). There are a number of barriers that prevent women from obtaining adequate STD care. Women in many cultures have little knowledge about their reproductive health and, therefore, few skills in diagnosing possible STD symptoms (Manneschmidt, see footnote 6). Pesce (1994) reported that several women in her study in Uruguay, especially poor women, had a complete lack of knowledge about their bodies and their sexuality.

As a result of shame, embarrassment, and the stigma associated with STDs, women are often reluctant to report to health services for the diagnosis and treatment of STDs. In many cultures, women have been socialized to feel shy about expressing anything in relation to their body that could be regarded as sexual (Tin Tin Saw 1995; Manneschmidt, see footnote 6). Also, many physicians are men, and there can be cultural barriers that prevent women from being seen by men who are not their husbands (Manneschmidt, see footnote 6).

Furthermore, because STDs are associated with "female deviance" and sexual immorality, some women may be highly concerned about the possibility of being ostracized by their family and their community (Guimarães 1994; Lwihula 1994). In contrast, STDs in males have become "a proud proof of manhood and virility" (Pinel 1994); consequently, there may be a higher level of reporting of STDs among men (Pinel 1994).

Care for STDs is generally restricted to STD clinics and women have reported that they were reluctant to use STD services because they felt uncomfortable attending clinics primarily frequented by prostitutes and men (Guimarães 1994). If they recognized the stigma associated with STDs, health services could improve the prospects that women would seek care by offering STD services in conjunction with primary health care and family-planning services. If the consultations were in privacy, it would not be obvious why the person was visiting the centre (Elias 1991; World Bank 1993).

Many health professionals reportedly lack knowledge about the symptoms of STDs, including AIDS (Guimarães 1994; Manneschmidt, see footnote 6). Furthermore, Guimarães (1994) pointed out that medical staff at a family-planning clinic in Brazil often ignored "minor" symptoms of STDs in female patients. Pesce (1994) reported that health-clinic professionals in Uruguay provided women with little or no information regarding the genesis of vaginal discharge, how it is transmitted, how it can be treated, or how it can be prevented. These findings suggest that more instruction on STDs, particularly from a gender perspective, is needed in the professional training of health providers.

Finally, in some cases there can be a requirement that infected individuals bring their partner as a condition for treatment, which may greatly affect compliance. Such stipulations should be eliminated. Individuals who are married or in permanent relationships and also have casual sexual partners may be unwilling to meet this condition (O'Connor et al. 1992; Lwihula 1994).

Chapter 5

The Working
Environment

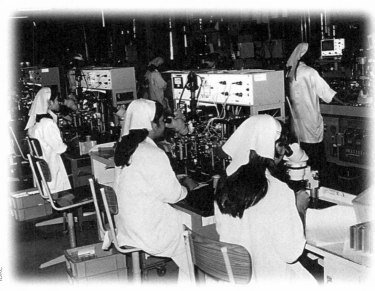

> Women constitute 50% of the world's population, do two-thirds
> of the world's work, and own one-tenth of the world's wealth.
> We are all raised in a culture that values men's work over
> women's work and men's lives over women's lives.
>
> — K. Soin, Member of Parliament, Singapore

Throughout the world, women work long and difficult hours in the formal and informal sectors, as well as in the household. However, in both industrialized and developing countries, the health implications of women's work is an area of study that has been relatively neglected (Messing 1991; Berr 1994; Haile 1994). According to Lee (1984, p. 15):

> Even in the developed countries where the occupational health movements are more established, very few studies have been done that focus on women's health. Among these, the majority focus on the reproductive health effects rather than the health of the women themselves.

As an example of the dearth of research on the health implications of women's work, Messing (1994) reported that a 1975–91 search of the Medline data bank for English-language studies that used the key words "dysmenorrhoea," "menstrual disorders," and "premenstrual tension" associated with "industry" or "occupation" or "worker" or "women," yielded no references in French or English, and one reference to a study written in Chinese relating occupational risk factors to menstrual symptoms. In addition to the lack of information on health issues commonly encountered in women's activities outside the home, there is also limited information showing the direct health effects of women's heavy workloads in the household (Messing 1991; Koblinsky, Campbell et al. 1993; Hatcher Roberts and Law 1994). According to Lee (1984, p. 15), a Malaysian researcher, "this lack of priority and interest [is] linked to the lowly status that society has accorded to women's work, particularly housework, which is seldom seen as being potentially hazardous."

Various health-related issues associated with women's work are addressed. A broad definition of "work" has been adopted, which includes not only wage-earning activities, but all activities whereby economic goods and services are produced and sold. The health risks associated with women's work in subsistence and domestic activities are also discussed.

There is a need for more research by government and nongovernment bodies in the occupational health and safety area. Practical tools need to be developed for the incorporation of occupational health and safety principles into the implementation, monitoring, and evaluation of government and nongovernment policies and programs. There is much ignorance and a scarcity of gender disaggregated data about women's actual roles, their work, and their important contribution to development. This workshop provides an ideal environment for sharing knowledge and experiences so that avenues to encourage research in this area, and bring visibility to the concerns of working women, can be explored.

— Ng Yen Yen, Senator to the Malaysian Parliament, Pahang, Malaysia

THE FORMAL WORK FORCE

In most regions around the world, women are playing an increasingly important role in the formally measured work force. This change in women's economic roles is creating additional health risks for women (Paolisso and Leslie 1995). Between 1950 and 1985, the number of economically active women in developing countries increased from 344 million to 675 million (Sivard 1985). According to the International Labour Organisation (ILO 1993), women represented over one-third of the global work force in the formal sector in 1990: 41.4% in the industrialized nations and 34.3% in the developing world.

In *Women's Lives and Women's Health*, Leslie (1992, p. 11) states that "While there are important variations among countries and over time, it is clear that the trend in the developing world has been an overall increase in women's participation in the paid labor force (including both informal and formal sector work)." This rapid expansion in market work for women is associated with a number of economic and social changes. These include: "increased monetization of economies, urbanization, declines in standards of living, improving educational attainment for women, and changes in social attitudes regarding the acceptability of women's participation in a broader economic world" (Paolisso and Leslie 1995, p. 61).

There are significant regional variations in women's formal work force participation rates. Figures in industrialized countries tend to be higher than in developing countries. In Canada, for example, 58% of Canadian women over age 15 years are in the paid labour force and comprise 45% of the total labour force (Status of Women Canada 1994).

In sub-Saharan Africa, women's share of the formal labour force in 1990 was 37% (UNDIESA 1991). Because most public and wage employees are men, women are invariably left to work in subsistence agriculture or to create whatever opportunities they can in the informal sector (UN 1991).

Female participation has increased in almost all Asian countries. According to official statistics, women's economic activity in southern and western Asia is very low (under 20%), but fairly high (35–40%) in eastern and southeastern Asia. In southeastern Asia, there has been significant expansion of economic opportunities for women. Female labour provides up to 80% of the work force of the export-producing zones (such as in the Republic of Korea and Thailand). However, women have usually been confined to repetitive assembly-line jobs in industries such as electronics, food processing, textiles, and footwear (ILO 1992a). Although more opportunities for women in the relatively advanced Asian economies reflect both women's higher educational status and growing labour shortages, in the low-income countries, increased women's participation, particularly in urban areas, is often related to poverty, and the need to increase household incomes (ILO 1994).

The changing social, political, and economic scenarios of many countries in the Asia–Pacific region has, and will continue to, radically change the role of women. As countries free themselves politically and economically and strive toward economic progress and development, an increasing number of women in the region will enter the work force.

— Ng Yen Yen, Senator to the Malaysian Parliament, Pahang, Malaysia

---

In Latin America, increased economic participation of women has also been observed. In Chile, for example, between 1970 and 1990, there was an 83% increase in the participation of women in the paid work force (Berr 1994). Formal work force participation rates for women are currently 31% in urban areas of Latin America and 14% in rural areas. Opportunities for women in urban areas have been closely tied to the greater economic necessities arising from the ongoing economic crisis of the 1980s. Low-income working women constitute an "invisible adjustment" to the economic crisis (UNICEF 1987).

Increased opportunities for women in some Latin American countries have also been related to women's higher educational attainment. One of the highest participation rates for females in the labour force in this region is in Uruguay (40%), which perhaps has the most successful secondary school system in the region (ILO 1994).

Continued growth in the Chilean economy will depend on the increasing incorporation of women into the labour force. However, the occupational health of the female worker is an area of research, and policy, that has thus far received little attention.

— Ximena Díaz Berr, Salaried Women in Industry and Fruitculture, Santiago, Chile

The service sector is particularly important in Latin America and employs about 70% of all economically active women, of which the highest proportion are in domestic service (ILO 1992a). In Brazil, for example, approximately one-third of the 15 million women who made up the female work force in 1985 were employed as domestic servants (Machado 1993).

THE INFORMAL WORK FORCE

Statistics focus only on the formally measured wage-earning participation of women in the labour force; they do not capture all the work done by women in the informal sector. When the health risks associated with women's work are addressed, it is crucial to recognize women's work in the informal sector, which is often missed by labour statistics. As described by Waring (1993, p. 109):

> Consider Tendai, a young girl in the Lowveld in Zimbabwe. Her day starts at 4:00 am when, to fetch water, she carries a 30 litre tin to a bore hole about 11 kilometres from her home. She walks bare foot and is home by 9:00 am. She eats a little and proceeds to fetch firewood until midday. She cleans the utensils from the family's morning meal and sits preparing a lunch of sudsa for the family. After lunch and the cleaning of the dishes, she walks in the hot sun until early evening, fetching wild vegetables for supper before making the evening trip for water. Her day ends at 9:00 pm after she's prepared supper and put her younger brothers to sleep. Tendai is considered unproductive, unoccupied and economically inactive. According to the International Economic System, Tendai does not work and is not part of the labour force.

Poor women hustle to make a living and put food in their children's mouths by working as wayside vendors, hucksters, suitcase traders, domestic workers, sex workers, and drug mules.

— Asha Kambon, Economic Commission for Latin America and the Caribbean, Port of Spain, Trinidad (see Kambon 1995)

Government statistics often omit much of the women's critical work that is useful to the continuing existence of the household, such as gathering fuel and water, raising a few animals, and keeping a kitchen garden (ILO 1985; Nuss 1989). The 1991 UNDIESA report, entitled *The World's Women*, states: "If women's unpaid work in subsistence agriculture and household and family care were fully counted in labour force statistics, their share of the labour force would be equal to or greater than men's."

In India, for example, official statistics suggest that 14% of the female population is working, compared with 52% of men. A special commission in 1988, however, found that more than 90% of working women in India were in the informal sector and unlikely to be recorded by the census-takers surveying the country's economy (Misch 1992).

Statistics overlook the increasing number of women worldwide who work as homeworkers and piece-workers, for example, weaving cloth, carpets, and baskets at home (Leslie 1992; Berr 1994; Haile 1994). Female street hawkers, such as the Andean peasants in Latin America who come from the country and from their indigenous communities to sell self-produced wares, food, and handicrafts in the cities, may also be ignored. According to Kambon (1995):

> High unemployment rates have pushed large segments of the female labour force into the informal sector ... as women in the Caribbean devise strategies to survive. Estimates are that between 30 and 50% of all employment is in the informal sector. In Guyana, ... the informal sector provides income for approximately 60% of the economy and in Haiti it is as high as 93%.

Much of women's activities are related to family occupations such as agriculture, animal husbandry, and forestry. These contributions of women, working without wages on family farms, may get merged with the family and become invisible, or viewed as "secondary, marginal, and supplementary."[11] Women may not report their agricultural labour as work despite the fact that during harvest season they can labour as many as 16 hours each day in the field (Khan and Midhet 1991, cited in Koblinsky, Timyan et al. 1993).

Although the International Labour Organisation (ILO) widened the definition of productive work in 1982 to include "all work for pay or in anticipation of profit" and "all production and processing of primarily products, whether for the market, for barter or for home consumption," the application of the new standard is far form universal, and in most countries, only a small part of women's production is measured. Survey investigators, often male, may not identify what women do as "work," but as part of their domestic

---

[11] See Mirdha, B.R., "The female client and the health provider." Unpublished paper submitted to the 1994–1995 TDR/IDRC competition.

responsibilities (Greenhalgh 1991; Nayak-Mukherjee 1991). Potential problems associated with collecting statistics on women's work in the Philippines were described by Illo (1991, p. 4).

> When collecting labor force or work data, census or statistics takers very often cursorily ask women what they do, to which countless women, particularly those in rural areas, respond "nothing." It should be noted that women's work, especially in the rural areas, consists of "small but many" enterprises .... The women consider all this as part and parcel of what being a good housewife ... means. The census taker, not trained to be sensitive to the nuances of people's own classificatory schemes, record countless women as "plain housewives" who, by definition, are "not working."

Women's work in the informal sector is repeatedly neglected despite the fact that it is frequently the only option for women and is crucial for their economic survival because they often cannot find work in the formal sector. As Greenhalgh (1991, p. 6) noted, "global processes of economic restructuring and labour deregulation have led to both an informalization and a feminization of the labour force in many parts of the world." Many women are in a situation where the husband — if there is one — is earning nothing, or not enough to guarantee a minimal basis of existence. The incomes of women in the informal sector become indispensable for the functioning of the household; as one women from Chad reported, "If I got a small scale trade, I could give my child what he needs; what his heart desires" (Wyss and Nandjingar 1995, p. 142).

THE SEXUAL DIVISION OF LABOUR

Throughout the world, there is a clear distinction between "women's work" and "men's work." According to Acevedo (1994), this differentiation originated in the sexual division of labour in the family and is perpetuated in the social organization of work outside the household. Men often have primary responsibility for tasks requiring heavy physical labour, such as cutting trees, hunting, the preparation of land for farming, and jobs that are specific to distant locations, such as livestock herding (Momsen 1991). In most cultures, the application of pesticides is considered a male task (Momsen 1991). Women, on the other hand, tend to be responsible for bearing children, caring for family members, and producing material goods that are directly consumed by the family, such as food and clothes (Acevedo 1994). In farming, "women carry out the repetitive, time consuming tasks like weeding, and those which are located close to home, such as the care of the kitchen garden" (Momsen 1991, p. 50).

In the work force, the sexual division of labour can be observed in the concentration of women in a narrow range of traditional or "female" occupations that tend to be poorly paid and lacking in status (ILO 1994). Women work in teaching, clerical work, sales, and domestic services, for example; whereas, men work in manufacturing, transportation, management, administration, and politics (UNDIESA 1991). This general pattern exists in industrialized countries, as well as developed nations. In Canada, in 1993, although women's participation in traditionally male-dominated professions had increased, 71% of all working women were employed in one of five occupational groups — teaching, nursing or related health occupations, clerical, sales, and services (Status of Women Canada 1994).

The sexual division of labour continues even when women and men work within the same industry, occupation, or profession. Men tend to be represented in the higher-ranking jobs, whereas women frequently work in low-skilled jobs and have little opportunity for advancement. In the textiles industry, for example, women work primarily as production workers and operators; in the electronics industries, women work on assembly lines; and in the garment industry, women work as tailors, sewing-machine operators, and clothes pressers. Furthermore, when an occupation or profession becomes predominantly "female," its economic and social status diminishes (ILO 1985).

WOMEN'S WORK AND ASSOCIATED HEALTH RISKS

Various types of women's work are examined along with selected health risks associated with these forms of work. Women's work in the agricultural sector, the service sector, and the industrial sector is examined first. Next, the health hazards linked to women's participation as homeworkers, a rapidly growing area, are reviewed. Finally, health risks associated with housework are explored in detail. Although these categories do not cover all varieties of women's work, they do encompass a major portion of the activities carried out by women in the developing world.

These categories of women's work are overlapping. For example, women's "housework" may include agricultural responsibilities. In addition, women employed in the industrial sector may perform their work at home and could, therefore, also be classified as homeworkers.

I am a worker, an organizer, a director, an administrator, an adviser, a doctor, a nurse, a cleaning woman, a gardener, a painter, a carpenter — you name it! I am the handyman, the jack of all trades.

— A black woman from northern KwaZulu-Natal, South Africa
(quoted in Pagé 1995, p. 8)

The agricultural sector

In many parts of the developing world, most women work in the agricultural sector — they work in both waged agricultural labour and subsistence agriculture. Their work can take the form of primary agriculture production, as well as processing, storage, and marketing of agricultural produce.

In sub-Saharan Africa, nearly 80% of economically active women are involved in agricultural labour (UNDIESA 1991). African women produce 80% of the food consumed domestically, and at least 50% of export crops (UNDIESA 1991). One study conducted by the Food and Agriculture Organization of the United Nations (FAO) reported that 80% of transporting and storing the harvest, 70% of the weeding and hoeing, and 50% of the sowing and planting are done by women (Haile 1994).

Although in many parts of Asia there has been a general shift in recent years to nonagricultural sectors of the economy (Nayak-Mukherjee 1991), the number of women involved in agriculture is still very high. Throughout southeastern Asia and the Indian subcontinent, at least 70% of the female labour force is engaged in agriculture (UNDIESA 1991). A study by ILO that detailed the way rural women spend their time indicated that up to 90% of rural women in central India participated in agriculture (Chatterjee 1990). More than 95% of economically active women work in agriculture in Bhutan and Nepal (UN 1991).

Despite these high participation rates, and the important contribution that women farmers make to the world's food supply, there is a dearth of good research that addresses the potential health risks associated with women's work in agriculture. The work of women may even be systematically ignored in research. For example, in Canada, Messing (1991) reported that female agriculture workers were excluded from a large ongoing study of cancer among farm operators, the "Mortality Study of Canadian Male Farm Operators," because the definition of "operator" used by Statistics Canada included only the farm owner, and women constituted less than 4% of this category.

We do know that women's agricultural work is arduous and tiring. The type of tasks that women perform — such as weeding, picking, and sorting

— means that they are at high risk of suffering injuries, backaches, severe arthritic pains, postural defects, and leg problems. The heavy and repetitive physical labour required in farm work is associated with musculoskeletal and soft tissue disorders and degenerative joint diseases of the hands, knees, and hips. Women agricultural workers in South India (Kerala and Tamil Nadu) who were involved in different stages of rice production reported that "they often made their children walk on their backs at night after a day's transplanting, in order to give them enough relief from pain so that they could go back and work the next day" (Mencher 1988, p. 104).

Women may have to work in the pouring rain as well as in the hot sun, with their feet deep in mud (Mencher 1988). Standing in water and mud all day while transplanting may lead to the splitting of the heels of the feet (Mencher 1988). Women may also be more readily exposed to a wide variety of infections and parasitic diseases (Mencher 1988; Chatterjee 1990).

Women's agricultural work is often carried out without the aid of labour-saving devices. Indeed, when agricultural technology — such as machines for land clearing, plowing, harvesting, and threshing — are introduced by development agencies, technology and related training may be exclusively provided to men (Butler et al. 1987, p. 20).

In the rice-growing industry [of Viet Nam], women have a number of responsibilities that are usually performed with rudimentary farm tools — plowing, sowing, transplanting, tending, weeding, and harvesting. Women in Viet Nam often spend 16 to 18 hours a day at work; whereas, men spend only 12 to 14 hours.

— Nguyen Thi Hoa Binh, Viet Nam Women's Union, Hanoi, Viet Nam (see Binh 1995)

In developing countries, pesticides are often misused, and health risks from excessive pesticide use may be increasing as women increasingly enter the growing agroexport sectors in many developing countries. Pesticides are absorbed through the skin, by inhalation, and by ingestion. Men, who are usually responsible for fumigating crops, may be exposed to high dosages of pesticides for short periods of time because of inadequate protection during application. *Strengthening Women*, a 1989 report from the International Center for Research on Women (ICRW), states:

> Women ... do more of the hand labor (such as weeding, picking and sorting) in fields that have been sprayed, thus encountering prolonged exposure to pesticides, [and] yet they usually wear little or no protective clothing. The threat of pesticide exposure has implications not only for a woman's own health, but also for that of their unborn and breastfed infants.

Although men are usually responsible for the application of pesticides, on Malaysian oil palm and cocoa plantations, "the sprayers who go on foot and manually spray the pesticides are almost always women (the men most often handle the spray trucks and other more sophisticated equipment). The pesticides used, such as paraquat, are poisonous if consumed and produce noxious fumes when sprayed; women report impaired eyesight, including blindness" (APDC 1992, p. 67).

Depending on the specific pesticide, exposure can cause neurological and behavioural problems, dermatitis, reproductive disorders, pulmonary problems, liver damage, eye damage (including corneal abrasion), and certain types of cancer (Enberg 1993). Women who work on Malaysian plantations have cited other effects of pesticides, such as dizziness, muscular pain, itching, skin burns, blisters, difficulty in breathing, nausea, changing nail colour, and sore eyes (Labour Resource Centre 1995).

Some agrochemicals have been linked to genetic defects in offspring. Spontaneous abortions, stillbirths, and premature births have also been attributed to certain chemicals used in agriculture (Messing 1991). Tragically, sometimes chemicals that have been banned in countries of origin or manufacture because of known adverse health effects are dumped for use in the developing world (Puta 1994).

In a study conducted by the Health Research and Consultancy Centre, 40% of female farmers in Sigchos, Ecuador, were found to have high levels of toxins in their blood. Chemicals used in agriculture (pesticides and fertilizers) got into women's blood systems through breathing and through skin contact and caused cancer, miscarriages, kidney problems, and headaches (MacMillan 1995).

In Chile, about 200 000 temporary workers, mostly women from 20 to 29 years of age, pick and pack fruit in Chile's booming agroexport industry that ships fruit all over the world. However, there is a darker side to Chile's fruit boom. One study showed that three times as many children were born with birth defects between 1988 and 1990 at a hospital located in a Chilean agricultural area (Rancagua Regional Hospital) than at the University of Santiago Clinical Hospital. The levels of spontaneous abortion were also particularly high at Rancagua: 211 per 1 000 pregnancies compared with 120 per 1 000 in Santiago (reported in Diebel 1995). The researcher, Victoria Mella, began her study after observing that an exceptionally high number of young women were aborting grotesquely deformed fetuses. As described by Diebel (1995, p. A18):

> The common denominator was that all had worked in the agricultural industry, often from the age of 12 .... [In Chile,] thousands of young women work away their childbearing years in pesticide-drenched fields, fearful that their babies will be born horribly deformed. They have no

protective clothing, no union, no government health standards to protect them .... All [the women] talk about the lack of protective clothing and masks, the contaminated drinking water, the constant coughs, allergies, bronchial problems, muscular spasms and dizziness.

Workers invariably are not properly informed of the many ill-effects associated with agrochemicals, and they may not be provided with protective clothing. In the flower-export industry in Ecuador, women, under pressure to meet production quotas, reportedly entered fields that had just been chemically treated, wearing no protective clothing or masks (Paolisso and Blumberg 1989). Women farmers in Ecuador "didn't know that clothes had to be washed to get rid of agricultural chemicals [if pesticides had been used]" (MacMillan 1995, p. 11).

If on-site washing facilities are unavailable, agricultural workers may eat their meals when their hands are still covered with pesticides from the crop they have been working on (Messing 1991). Lack of knowledge about the dangers of pesticides means that unsuspecting workers often use discarded containers contaminated with pesticides to store drinking water (LaDou 1993).

The processing of agricultural products may also have harmful health effects. For example, in Brazil, Mozambique, and Sri Lanka, cashew nuts are produced for export and women process the crop. This involves removing the nut from its protective outer casting that contains an acid that can harm the skin if protective clothing is not worn (Momsen 1991). In the preparation of cassava, a major food crop throughout tropical Africa and in many Pacific countries, a deadly poison — hydrogen cyanide — is released. Women, predominantly responsible for processing cassava, may be exposed to hydrogen cyanide fumes during their work and suffer related health effects (Ferrar 1992).

Women make up a large part of the tobacco-growing work forces in many developing nations. They work in the fields and processing plants. In Indonesia, cigarette manufacturers employ about 15 million people, mostly women. In Brazil, women strip tobacco from its stems in warehouses where the humidity and smell from the tobacco can cause headaches, vomiting, dizziness, and shortness of breath (Greaves et al. 1994). Further research on the impact of tobacco growing on women's health is urgently required.

It should be noted that illnesses related to women's working environment, whether they result from women's participation in agriculture or from other types of women's work, may be exacerbated by a number of factors related to the general health and well-being of women. For example, poor nutrition and lack of sufficient rest, often associated with poverty, may increase the effects of workplace illness (Haile 1994; Puta 1994). As Messing (1991, p. 10) pointed out: "The healthy young body may resist damage from workplace chemicals better than the unhealthy or older body ... the poorly nourished body may be less able to tolerate polluted air."

Furthermore, infections and parasitic diseases that are not necessarily related to occupation, for example, malaria, hookworm, and AIDS, may aggravate the effects of illness or disease associated with women's work.

The service sector

Services form an important sector of employment for women. Service-sector employment includes work in nursing, secretarial, teaching, sales, and catering work. Women also work in restaurants and hotels and perform domestic labour. These types of activities are thought to be "typically female," because they are perceived to be an extension of women's traditional roles.

In Latin America and the Caribbean, 71% of economically active women are involved in the service sector. In Asia, 40% of women are employed in the service sector. However, in Africa, only 20% of women counted as economically active work in this sector (UNDIESA 1991).

Women [in Venezuela] are concentrated in the so-called "female ghettos." For example, twice as many women than men work in the service area, such as restaurants, hotels, and domestic labour.

— Doris Acevedo, Carabodo University, Maracay, Venezuela

Characteristics of work in the service sector, one of the so-called "female ghettos" (Acevedo 1994), include minimal decision-making and working with the public. Although dealing with the public and responding to the needs of others can be rewarding, it can also be very demanding and difficult (Messing 1991) and lead to high stress levels, exhaustion, and a state of burnout. Excessive stress increases the risk of workplace accidents, as well as the chance of developing cardiovascular disease (Lowe 1989). These jobs involve monotonous tasks, minimal creativity, and little control over the external environment, all of which may contribute to mental health problems (Acevedo 1994).

An increased need for female domestic workers, to perform child care and other domestic responsibilities, has developed in some parts of the world as more and more women take full-time paid employment outside the home. As a result, a growing number of domestic workers from developing countries are migrating to industrialized countries.[12] These women may experience

---

[12] Such as from the Philippines and Caribbean countries to Canada and from the Philippines to Hong Kong and Singapore.

"emotional torment of leaving families behind, as well as difficult working conditions, job insecurity and potential employer abuse" (Grandea 1994, p. 13).

Women from Bangladesh, India, the Philippines, and Sri Lanka are lured to countries such as Kuwait, Saudi Arabia, and the United Arab Emirates to work as "virtual slave for prosperous Arab families" (Serrill 1995, p. 57). Serrill continues (p. 57):

> It is common for the maids to be forced to work from dawn to midnight, seven days a week. Often they are fed scraps and lefovers, and beaten and verbally abused and, in the worst cases, raped and murdered. Only in the most egregious instances is the employer ever charged with sexual abuse or assault.

As well, as reported by Dickson (1995):

> Domestic workers are exposed to the multiple risks of the home environment where most accidents occur. These include exposure to poisons in pesticides and cleaning materials, high risk of falls, long hours on their feet, frequent expectations to work overtime and on holidays, which deprives their own families. All this is often for inadequate remuneration. In this era of increasing opportunity, many women have opted out of being full-time housekeepers, but yet have not necessarily improved conditions for their proxies.

The health problems and working conditions of middle education teachers in the state of Maracay in Venezuela (about 75% of whom are women) were explored by Acevedo (1994). A review of medical records of the educators found that the most common health complaints were depression, arterial tension problems, and voice problems. The most frequent causes of absence from work were depression, anxiety, recurring headaches, functional diaphony, nodules on vocal cords, and high blood pressure. Acevedo pointed out that these disorders were related to the specific conditions of teaching: work with the public; an intensive working day; excessive use of the voice; low salary; and low social prestige.

In many countries, women constitute up to 75% of the labour force in the health sector (Jones and Catalan 1989; Strebel 1994; Lule and Ssembatya 1995). However, the majority of the better paid, more prestigious and authoritative positions as medical physicians and managers, continue to be held by men. Women, on the other hand, tend to fill the lower status, poorly paid (or unpaid), but nevertheless crucial, roles as nurses, midwives, auxiliaries and community health workers, and traditional birth attendants.

Women comprise the vast majority of volunteers in hospitals, self-help clinics, and other community health organizations despite their already significant workloads within the household (Lange et al. 1994). Indeed, the success of primary health-care programs and child-survival strategies has largely depended on women's involvement (Leslie et al. 1988; Kwawu 1994). Women perform vital and multiple tasks such as: providing health education to mothers about the importance of prenatal care, good diet during pregnancy, breastfeeding, proper weaning, immunizations, and management of diarrhea; monitoring the growth of infants and young children; distributing oral rehydration therapy; providing simple treatment and referrals; providing social and emotional support to community members; monitoring blood pressure; helping others to make decisions about when to go to health services and making appointments for those who need assistance; and participating in various prevention campaigns (World Bank 1993; Lange et al. 1994). Female traditional birth attendants deliver most of the babies in the developing world.

In Laos, for example (Boupha 1995):

> Led by the Lao Women's Union members, Lao women, as grandmothers, mothers, daughters, nieces, aunts, and neighbours, play a great role in the family and in the community by providing health education .... They are bringing to the community an awareness of the importance of child immunization and knowledge about such things as sanitary activities, family planning, contraception, and methods of birth spacing.

The enthusiasm and willingness of women to work as volunteer health providers is consistent with prescribed gender expectations and stereotypes. According to socially defined duties and expectations, women are expected to serve, nurture, and understand others, to do so quietly without expecting praise, to never refuse requests made by others, and to be unconcerned with monetary compensation (Lange et al. 1994). Indeed, in the study by Lange et al. (1994) of female health providers in Santiago, Chile, over half of the women interviewed did not expect any economic compensation for their work. They emphasized that they were proud that their work was voluntary, and that payment would serve to lessen its value. Providers who indicated

---

We learned [in the program] that health is very important, that we have to learn many things, not learning how to treat illnesses, but how to prevent them. The program helped me a lot, because as a person, although I am still a little shy, I already speak to others and we deal with each other, we feel like equals. It is nice to deal with people of the community, to go and teach them. Sometimes we are welcomed, sometimes we are not, but at the end they understand what we are teaching them.

— A participant in an education and development program in primary health care in Colombia. (quoted in Collazos V. 1994)

that they would like to be paid said that they would use the money to reduce the expenses incurred in performing their work or to buy implements necessary for their work.

Although not the primary objective of health programs, women's involvement in primary health-care programs often contributes to the personal development of individual women and leads to immense satisfaction. In the study by Lange et al. (1994) of volunteer health-care workers in Chile, women were motivated to do this work because of the expectation of personal development, which could be attained through training, and the perception that the work represented an opportunity to do something useful for the community. Women said that their work allowed them to establish positive relationships with members of their community and gave them an opportunity to help others, which made them feel positive, helped them make good use of their time, and enriched their development as human beings. Training helped them feel more self-reliant and better able to face certain daily situations. For example, some women stated that, prior to being health-care workers, they did not feel confident to speak in public or to discuss issues with physicians or other health professionals. Training increased their self-esteem and their capacity to undertake important tasks (Lange et al. 1994).

> Women's contribution [as health providers] is undervalued and women become discouraged by the lack of recognition they receive. Women risk being perceived and treated as resources that can be drawn on until exhausted.
>
> — Ilta Lange, School of Nursing, Universidad Católica de Chile, Santiago, Chile

Although women can gain much satisfaction from their role as health providers, women may also experience a sense of frustration and discouragement because the value of their contribution is not fully recognized. This lack of recognition can negatively affect the stability, continuity, and effectiveness of their work (Lange et al. 1994). In their study, when women were asked what they disliked most about their community "voluntary work," 75% pointed out elements related to the way other people reacted to their wish to help. They mentioned apathy, lack of cooperation, criticism, ungratefulness, and the fact that their work was not recognized by the community they were serving (Lange et al. 1994).

Likewise, in Bangladesh, traditional birth attendants or *dai*, reported that they did not receive sufficient recognition from families for their services. For example, even though *dai* are widely recognized as experienced women whose presence is desired at a birth, they sometimes did not receive a cash payment, or a suitable substitute for cash, such as a sari, after the child was delivered. The following comment was typical: "When in danger, they call you, but when the danger in over, get lost" (Rozario 1995, p. 95). In contrast, an attending doctor always received a substantial fee, even when it was the *dai* who actually delivered the baby while the doctor stood by. Despite this lack of gratitude, traditional birth attendants said they would continue to help families who asked for their assistance (Rozario 1995).

Because of the valuable, and largely voluntary role that female health providers play, there is a risk that health services may place onerous demands on women. Increased reductions in state-supported health-care programs mean further burdens for women. In addition, because of the way women have been socialized, they may not complain about such adverse conditions. Efforts are needed to ensure that female health providers are not exploited and that their work is fully acknowledged (Lange et al. 1994).

The industrial sector

Women's participation in the industrial labour force of many developing countries has risen over the past two decades. In newly industrialized economies such as Hong Kong, Singapore, South Korea, and Taiwan, and in others such as Malaysia, Mexico, the Philippines, Thailand, and some of the Caribbean countries, women have increasingly taken jobs in factories and, therefore, been exposed to new occupational risks (Vickers 1991; Jacobson 1993).

Some developing countries have set up economic production zones or free trade zones that offer various incentives, such as attractive tax packages and a cheap, well-disciplined, manually dextrous and highly productive work force, to encourage multinational corporations to set up production (Nayak-Mukherjee 1991; Vickers 1991). Some governments have attempted to increase their nations' comparative advantage by waiving worker-protection legislation that increases labour costs (LaDou 1993). The Malaysian government advertised "cheap, docile, highly trainable, non-unionized labour," to attract foreign investment (Lim 1988, p. 37). In the free-trade zones of Southeast and South Asia, the workers in the labour-intensive manufacturing of electronics, textiles, and footwear are predominantly female (75–90%), single, and young (15–29 years) (Nayak-Mukherjee 1991; Yen 1995). "Many authors have forcefully argued that the dynamism and economic growth witnessed in the economies of South-East Asian countries have been achieved largely due to the female-participation, as the sectors that have been crucial frontiers of growth have also been the sectors with female-dominated work force" (Nayak-Mukherjee 1991, p. 16).

> Girls and young women are a particular target in a highly
> competitive climate where they are seen as a source of cheap,
> docile labour; easy to hire and easy to fire when they are no
> longer needed. Tens of thousands of young girls are working in
> factories, using tools designed for adults, carrying heavy loads,
> and working long hours with no breaks and few, if any, safety
> standards to protect them.
>
> — A. El Bindari Hammad, World Health Organization, Geneva, Switzerland

The working conditions in these factories are frequently abysmal. Women can usually only obtain the lowest-skilled, lowest-paid jobs because of lack of education and training opportunities (Vickers 1991) and systemic discrimination on the basis of sex. Women commonly work in unregulated industries that may be outside the scope of occupational health and safety legislation or trade unions (ILO 1985; World Bank 1993). Some firms reportedly restrict the number of years that they employ individual women to prevent the build up of senior workers who may demand higher wages (ILO 1985; Nayak-Mukherjee 1991). Other plants control the women's lives 24 hours a day by housing them in dormitory accommodations.

Considerable stress is associated with this type of factory employment. Female workers habitually face extremely high productivity targets, can work 7 days a week at monotonous tasks, and work odd shift hours. Factory employees working at piecework rates, or paid by the hour, are subject to extreme time pressures, which may result in anxiety and stress. A fast work pace may cause workers to neglect important safety precautions, which can increase the risk of accidents (Messing 1991).

An insecure employment situation, in which women can lose their jobs during production cutbacks or when firms relocate in search for new sources of cheap labour, further compounds stress levels. According to Nayak-Mukherjee (1991), a relocation of industries has been noticed from Singapore to Indonesia, Malaysia, Thailand and from there to Sri Lanka and very recently, to Bangladesh and even China. Not surprisingly, these stressful conditions may result in migraines, nervous breakdowns, and "burn-out" (Nayak-Mukherjee 1991).

Other unhealthy working conditions in the industrial sector include poor ventilation, inadequate lighting, heat, humidity, radiation, and overcrowding, which may affect physical health and decrease productivity (Soin 1995). Noise, an extremely frequent problem in factories (World Bank 1993; Puta 1994), can result in industrial deafness, and is also a major stress factor for workers (Messing 1991). Facilities for women, such as toilets, may be inadequate. For example, in one typical factory in Bangladesh, where over 200 women and 50 men were working, there was only one toilet for women and one for men (Hossain and Sobhan 1988).

Indoor air pollution may lead to discomfort, headaches, and respiratory problems (Messing 1991). The harmful effects of high dust concentrations on workers' health, especially on their respiratory systems, is a well-known fact in the field of occupational health (Carasco 1994; Haile 1994). As well as respiratory-tract difficulties, dust has been found to have significant associations with accidents, general illness, and absence (Meng et al. 1987).

Results from a study carried out at the National Institute of Occupational and Environmental Health in Hanoi, Viet Nam (Nga 1995), showed the following.

> Women workers were exposed to hazardous agents in the workplace such as heat, toxic gases, noise, dust, and chemicals .... Characteristics of work in industries with new imported technologies included the monotonous motion of small muscle groups, poor air quality in working rooms ... and a significant difference in indoor and outdoor temperatures.

Women, stereotypically perceived as passive, predominate in jobs that require prolonged standing or sitting, often in uncomfortable positions, and in seats that are not ergonomically designed. Muscular pain, including back pain, and neck, shoulder, and leg problems, are health issues associated with static work (Acevedo 1994; Haile 1994). Prolonged standing, without moving, may strain the musculoskeletal system and interfere with blood circulation to and from the legs, which can lead to leg pain, cramps, numbness, and swelling in the lower legs and feet (Corlett and Bishop 1976; Waterfield 1981; Messing 1991).

Although some hazards are obvious, others are insidious and slow to manifest themselves. Workers may be exposed to dust-laden air, to fumes and gases in chemical extraction plants, to artificial humidification in cotton mills, to paints and solvents that can be absorbed through the skin. Their work on conveyor belt production may be boring and tedious.

— Anne Kamoto Puta, Zambian Organization of Occupational Health and Safety, Zambia

> More than half of the medical problems were of a respiratory
> nature. This was related to the high dust concentration in the
> textile factory.
>
> — Joseph Carasco, Centre for Basic Research, Kampala, Uganda

Textile workers

Among predominantly female textile and garment workers, byssinosis, or
"brown lung," is a common occupational lung disease of workers who process
cotton and are exposed to raw cotton dust. Its symptoms include breathless-
ness and tightness of the chest, and it can lead to chronic bronchitis or
emphysema (Committee of Asian Women 1987; Labour Resource Centre
1995; Paolisso and Leslie 1995).

Textile workers may be exposed to harmful chemicals and may be
unaware of the possible toxic effects of the chemical materials that they handle (Puta 1994). Exposure to chemicals used for dyeing, bleaching, and making fabrics shrink-resistant can lead to eye irritations, sore throat, allergic
reactions, and skin rashes (Committee of Asian Women 1987).

The operation of a sewing machine requires repetitive movements of
fingers, wrists, and elbows at high speeds (APDC 1990; Vézina et al. 1992),
can cause extreme and persistent pain, and may eventually result in neurological and musculoskeletal problems such as bursitis, epicondylitis, carpal
tunnel syndrome, and tenosynovitis of the wrist (Kurppa et al. 1979; Punnet
1985; Messing 1991). Garment workers are prone to accidents such as sewing
needles piercing fingers, which tends to occur when fast work under stressful
conditions is required (Committee of Asian Women 1987). Sewing machin-
ists may also experience high levels of backache, neckache, and shoulder and
elbow problems (Messing 1991; Rowbotham 1993). One women who had
worked at a sewing machine for several years reported that "the consequences to my health cannot be compared. My hands were tired all the time.
I could not use them for heavy work, and if I did, they would hurt"
(Rowbotham 1993, p. 40).

This type of work, like much of women's work, is boring, repetitive,
and monotonous. It also offers little opportunity for communication with
others. The effects of these workplace conditions on the minds and general
health of workers has not been well documented (Messing 1991; Acevedo
1994).

Textile workers may also be exposed to dangerous machinery (Berr
1994; Carasco 1994), have no protective devices, and not receive the

training necessary for safe use. Women textile workers in Ethiopia, for instance, routinely work without protective devices (Haile 1994).

Electronics workers

Like the textiles industry, the electronics industry predominantly employs women. In the Malaysian electronics industry, for example, 85% of the employment is female — and 92% of these jobs are unskilled. And, in Malaysia, "the concentration of women in electronics is no mere coincidence ... the presence of a large, low-wage, female work force is a well-documented reason for corporate decisions to locate [there]" (Labour Resource Centre 1995).

The main reported health hazard associated with women's work in electronics is related to eye damage. Female electronic workers on semiconductor assembly lines "using microscopes the whole day to join tiny wires to semiconductor chips" (APDC 1990, p. 18), often suffer from eyestrain that can result in conjunctivitis, nearsightedness, deteriorating eyesight, and double vision (APDC 1990; Nayak-Mukherjee 1991).

In addition, a range of potentially hazardous chemicals may be used in various stages of the electronics assembly process, including trichloroethylene (TCE), methyl ethyl ketone (MEK), xylene, acetone, solder flux, sulfuric acid, and hydrochloric acid. Exposure to these chemicals has been linked to skin and respiratory diseases and to spontaneous abortions (Labour Resource Centre 1995; Yen 1995).

Homeworkers

The specific health concerns of homeworkers warrant attention because nearly all homeworkers are women and homeworkers make up an integral part of the informal economy in most developing nations. "Homework," by definition, is the production of a good or the provision of a service, for an employer or contractor, at a place of the worker's own choosing, often the worker's own home, usually without direct supervision by the employer or the contractor. Homeworkers are also referred to as "outworkers," "home-based workers," or "piece-rate workers" (ILO 1992b, p. 3).

It is difficult to ascertain the actual numbers of homeworkers because they are unlikely to be recorded by statistics; however, the ILO has estimated that homeworkers account for between 5% and 35% of the gross domestic product in several developing countries for which it has gathered data (Misch 1992). Homeworkers are increasingly developing into a large international "shadow economy" in most industrialized and developing countries. As manufacturers respond to international competition by fragmenting their production process, they increasingly rely on routine work done by women in their own homes (Messing 1991). Homeworkers are "weaving carpets in Turkey, stitching shoes in Italy, making garments in the United States, laundering clothes in Ecuador, and assembling metal dish-washing sponges in Mexico" (Misch 1992, p. 18).

The types of work that homeworkers perform in developing countries is extremely wide-ranging: homeworkers are involved in the production of clothing, textiles, tobacco, carpets and rugs, and wicker and leather works (ILO 1992b); they perform ancillary tasks such as sorting, cleaning, packaging, and labelling; and they may engage is the subassembly of electrical and electronic products, as well as working in traditional industries associated with the preparation of food, handicrafts, and pottery (Haile 1994).

On the surface, home-based work offers some advantages to women. Because homeworkers tend to be married women who have children and only a primary education (ILO 1992b), homework provides these women, who are often living in poverty, with the opportunity to earn some income while they attend to their children and other household responsibilities (ILO 1992b, 1994).

Although little is known about the working conditions of homework-ers because of the lack of documentation, the available information suggests that conditions are typically very poor. Homework usually involves very long hours, which may lead to extreme fatigue. Extremely low pay for piece work encourages women to work extra long hours. In India, for example, women may role cigarettes from before dawn until long past dusk. According to one tobacco roller: "My days start at 5:30 in the morning and end at 11:30 at night. My life started with the rolling of beedis [cigarettes] and perhaps it will end that way too" (Misch 1992, p. 18).

Homeworkers face many of the same problems as women who work in other sectors. For example, like much of women's work, homework is typi-cally repetitive, monotonous, and lacking in variety. Homeworkers, such as Indian bangel workers and lace-makers, may suffer from eye disorders because of the fine detail demanded by their handiwork (Misch 1992). Tobacco workers may experience "arms swollen from cutting, and asthma from breathing tobacco dust" (Misch 1992, p. 18). A survey of homeworkers in the garment industry carried out by the Self-Employed Women's Association (SENA) in Gujarat, India, in 1986 found that 90% of the women complained of pain in the feet and legs; 82% reported back pain; 31% suf-fered from pain in their hands. Headaches, abdominal pain, and eyestrain were other common complaints. Homeworkers can suffer from accidents related to their homework, such as injuries from knife cuts and the piercing of fingers by needles (ILO 1992b).

Factors that distinguish homework from other forms of work create additional hazards for the health and well-being of women. Because homeworkers are not registered as workers, and they do not work under fixed contracts, their employers generally take no responsibility for their health and security (Misch 1992). As Misch (1992, p. 19) stated, they are "beyond the reach of those laws and regulations that offer workers some measure of protection from exploitation." A Malaysian homeworker who worked until after midnight most evenings making paper "money" used in Chinese funeral ceremonies said, "I worry that I have no sickness or unemployment protection, and I often get backaches and sore eyes" (Mitter 1986, p. 119).

> *Being generally excluded from secure and bargainable jobs in the formal sector, women are willing to accept employment that offers them a livelihood, however insecure.*
>
> — Swasti Mitter, Institute for New Technologies, United Nations University, Maastricht, Netherlands (see Mitter 1994)

Homeworkers are also isolated from fellow workers (Messing 1991) and have no access to channels such as trade unions for wage bargaining and the articulation of health-related concerns. In addition, because it is unlikely that their homes have been equipped or designed properly for the required task, homeworkers may, for example, work in highly uncomfortable working positions or have inadequate ventilation (Johnson 1982). Finally, Messing (1991, p. 13) pointed out that because "children may be present at the worksite, women may be required to divide their concentration between child care and the task at hand, thus increasing the risk of accidents for both themselves and their children" (Messing 1991, p. 13).

Housework

In addition to women's participation in the work process through their work in the formal and informal sectors, women also participate through their work at home (Acevedo 1994). Women in all societies tend to have significant responsibilities within the household. The numerous domestic tasks usually carried out by women include preparing food for the family over smoky fires in unventilated kitchens; caring for family members including children, the sick, and the elderly; providing food, firewood, and water for home consumption; carrying heavy loads over long distances; educating and supervising children; looking after the upkeep of the home; and tending the kitchen garden and livestock. It is clear, as Wyss and Nandjingar (1995,

> *Nowhere is "housework" defined, so that it becomes the generic term for everything that women do in an unpaid capacity.*
>
> — Waring (1993, p. 109).

p. 142) pointed out, that "a housewife does not lack work." In the words of Cardaci (1992):

> As a provider, the woman is responsible for guaranteeing ... a safe atmos-phere: a warm and clean house where family members are protected from illnesses and dangers, where children, young people, and adults are offered a balanced diet .... It is a woman's role to maintain family har-mony inside a home and to diminish the anxieties and tensions that emerge when these relationships do not go well. Home as a refuge ... is "typically" a woman's responsibility.

Although women are increasingly entering the paid work force, this has not led to the lessening of household burdens. Instead, women feel responsible for doing both home and work-related jobs efficiently, and often this means that it is done at the expense of women's own health and well-being.

Household labour, central to the maintenance of social systems, is not compensated by society in monetary terms. Because "work" if often viewed as "paid activity," the important but unpaid work of women at home tends to be overshadowed and marginalized (Berr 1994). However, by their labour in the household, women are subsidizing the production and maintenance of the work force.

Because many women work in the home, they suffer disproportion-ately from the health risks in the household environment. Although many of the traditional responsibilities of women make them more susceptible to specific health effects, "very little research has been done to investigate the prevalence of these health conditions, their importance to women, their impact on productivity and well-being, or on how to alleviate them" (Vlassoff 1994, p. 1251).

National and international statistics about women's economic roles tend to completely ignore the work done by women within the household (Rathgeber 1994a). However, if housework is taken into account when mea-suring women's work, women work much longer hours than men in most parts of the world (ILO 1992a; Acevedo 1994) (Figure 4). Research must explicitly incorporate women's unpaid housework into the conceptualization and measurement of women's work activities.

Indoor air pollution

According to the World Bank (1993), indoor air pollution probably exposes more people worldwide to important air pollutants than does pollution in outdoor air. Women throughout the developing world are predominantly responsible for the cooking of food, and they, as well as their young children, suffer the greatest exposure.

Furthermore, the WHO estimates that about half of the world's population uses biomass (such as wood and cow dung) as cooking and heating fuel, often without proper ventilation. In India, for example, 99% of rural households and more than 50% of urban households use biomass cooking fuels (APDC 1990). Proximity to indoor household stoves that use biomass fuels has been linked to acute respiratory infections in young children and to

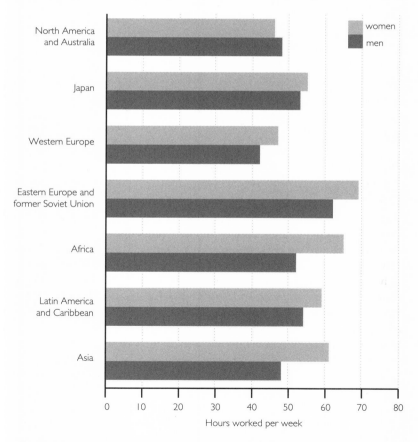

Figure 4. Total amount of work time for women and men (including housework) in 1990 (source: UNDIESA 1991).

chronic lung diseases and cancer in adults. Exposure during pregnancy may also lead to adverse pregnancy outcomes, such as stillbirths, right-side heart failure, and low birthweight (World Bank 1993; Haile 1994). Women may also suffer daily discomforts such as irritated eyes, running noses, and headaches.

Because women are closely associated with domestic duties, they are more affected by pollutants in the household caused by the use of fuels such as kerosene and industrial byproducts such as rubber, canvas, leather, oil seed cakes, and fuelwood. These factors contribute to the high incidence of asthmatic and other respiratory diseases, as well as eye problems.

— Fekerte Haile, International Labour Organisation, Addis Ababa, Ethiopia

---

Studies in China, India, Nepal, and Papua New Guinea have shown that up to half of adult women (few of whom smoke) suffer from chronic lung and heart disease because of the high levels of indoor smoke. Nonsmoking Chinese women exposed to indoor coal smoke (which is especially harmful) have a risk of lung cancer similar to that of men who smoke lightly (World Bank 1993).

A study of four villages in rural Gujarat, India, found that women who cooked in poorly ventilated huts were exposed, on average, to 100 times the level of suspended smoke particles deemed acceptable by the WHO, six times higher levels than other household members, and 15 times higher than a resident of Delhi (Chatterjee 1990). Another study in India estimated that while women were cooking they inhaled as much of the carcinogen benzopyrene as if they smoked 20 packs of cigarettes a day (WHO 1984). In the high-altitude mountain areas of Nepal, women often suffer from a disease similar to anemia. The illness is caused by carbon monoxide in the bloodstream, the result of long-term exposure to the pollutants from crude energy sources such as indoor cooking fires (Easterbrook 1994). Acute respiratory infections and chronic bronchitis are also very common in rural areas of India and Nepal as a result of exposure to kitchen smoke (UN 1995).

Paolisso (1995) suggested that deforestation and fuelwood scarcity may increase health risks for women from smoke pollution because they are forced to use lower quality, quick-burning biomass fuels, which increase the time spent tending cooking fires. He pointed out, however, that there is little documentation of the extent to which fuel substitution is occurring, nor any reliable evidence of its health implications.

There is clearly an urgent need for more research on the health effects of this common activity. In addition, the extent to which modifications to home cooking and heating facilities — such as stove design, ventilation design, and fuel type — would reduce exposure to the detrimental effects of indoor air pollution needs to be explored. However, efforts to reduce indoor smoke levels may increase the biting activity of insect vectors in malaria-endemic communities because smoke repels the insects. Therefore, interventions aimed at reducing household smoke in malaria-endemic regions should be coupled with malaria-control interventions, such as pesticide-impregnated bednets.

Tropical diseases

Depending on the sexual division of labour, women's household responsibilities and culturally prescribed roles can also increase their exposure to waterborne diseases such as schistosomiasis. For example, in communities where women are responsible for washing clothes and laundry or cleaning kitchen utensils through immersion or partial immersion in infected waters, women may have higher infection rates than men during peak periods of cercarial shedding (Huang and Manderson 1992; Anyangwe et al. 1994). Furthermore, women who work or travel to get fuel and fodder from areas where open-field defecation is practiced risk exposure to diseases that can be spread via human excrement (such as typhoid, amoebic dysentery, parasitic infections, and hookworm).

Heavy weights

Many of the traditional responsibilities of women in the developing world are load-associated: women often carry, lift, and transport heavy loads in their daily activities. For example, the responsibility of obtaining fresh water for drinking, cooking, cleanliness, and hygiene, often from long distances in heavy containers, is almost exclusively that of women and girls (Carasco 1994; Hatcher Roberts and Law 1994). Small-scale studies in Asia and Africa indicate that women and girls spend an average of 5–17 hours per week collecting and carrying water (UN 1991). However, Butler et al. (1987) reported that when the trip to a water source is facilitated by other means of transport (such as a bicycle, donkey, wheelbarrow, or oxcart), some men may become involved.

As well, Rosina Wiltshire remarked that "water pumps that have been installed in many communities have proven to be useless. Although women tend to be responsible for water collection, these pumps have primarily been designed and located for use by men."

> *Young girls and women in Ethiopia frequently carry up to 77 kilograms of fuelwood and other produce, and travel an average of 11 or 12 kilometres daily.*
>
> — Fekerte Haile, International Labour Organisation, Addis Ababa, Ethiopia

Women are also responsible for obtaining fuelwood. Gurinder Shahi of the United Nations Development Programme (UNDP) estimated that, in Nepal, rural women spend 5 or 6 hours a day on foot searching for fuelwood and carrying it home (Easterbrook 1994). Young girls and women in Ethiopia frequently carry up to 77 kilograms of fuelwood and other produce, and travel an average of 11–12 kilometres daily (Haile 1985; Abegaz and Junge 1990). In Table 3, load data for fuelwood carriers in Ethiopia are compared with ILO weight limits.

Carrying heavy loads over long distances is physically demanding and exhausting work. In addition to fatigue, heavy weights can cause an increased incidence of back strains, lower-back pain, fractures, chronic and debilitating back and leg problems, damage to the knees, and other physical damage (ILO 1989; Haile 1994). In Viet Nam, for example, heavy physical work is common and "loads carried on the head were found to have a detrimental effect on the vertebrae of workers (especially in the neck region)" (Nga 1995).

Water is carried on the head, the back, the shoulder, or the hip, depending on the region of the world (APDC 1990), and each method may create health problems for women. Women who carry water on their back often walk in a stooped position. Asymmetric shoulder carrying may cause the body to develop more on one side. Hip damage can result from carrying water on the hip (APDC 1990), and the carrying of water on the back using a head strap may lead to severe headaches.

Table 3. ILO limits for loads to be lifted and carried by women compared with loads commonly lifted and carried in Ethiopia.

Age (years)	Permissible loads (kg) Occasionally[a]	Frequently[b]	Average load (kg) lifted and carried by women in Ethiopia
15–18	15	10	46
19–45	15	10	64
Over 45	15	10	55

Source: ILO (1989), Haile (1994).
[a] Limits that cannot be exceeded without health risk.
[b] Values recommended from an ergonomic point of view.

Carrying heavy loads, such as large containers of water, can also lead to a prolapsed uterus (Labour Resource Centre 1995) and is associated with menstrual disorders, miscarriage, and stillbirth (NCSEW 1988). Girls who begin carrying heavy loads of water at a young age are at risk for scoliosis (Chatterjee 1991).

The Asian and Pacific Development Centre (APDC 1990, p. 112) also points out that women are exposed to skeletal problems, which could lead to deformity and disability.

> One of these is damage to the vertebral column (spine) which due to overwork can degenerate and lead to arthrosis, a degenerative rheumatism or cyphosis (a permanently bent back). Pain is constant and mobility becomes less until a stage may be reached where people cannot move at all.

In older working women in the developing world, researchers report that functional disability is most strongly related to years spent fetching water (Doty 1987). This type of physical damage can in turn increase the burden of women's work.

Environmental degradation and women's workloads

Because women are closely tied to natural resources, environmental degradation can have a immediate and dramatic impact on women's workloads and livelihoods, as well as on the health and living conditions of the family as a whole (Muntemba 1989; Soin 1995). Environmental degradation includes negative changes to the physical environment and the ecology, such as water pollution, receding vegetation, destroyed forests, and poor soils (Tsikata 1994).

If environmental degradation decreases the amount of food produced by the land and waters, or diminishes the availability of fuel to cook meals, women, who are largely responsible for feeding their families, become

---

Land clearing and timber cutting causes deforestation and this forces rural women to search further from home for fuelwood. Deforestation then causes the loss of ground water, and the use of pesticides and fertilizers further damages water resources and leads then to shortages of water for domestic use. This impacts on the health and living conditions of the family, and the women are exhausted in their search for water and fuel.

— K. Soin, Member of Parliament, Republic of Singapore

exhausted as they are forced to work longer hours to make ends meet (Jacobson 1992a). A study in rural Kenya found that agricultural marginalization and environmental deterioration were increasing the work burdens of women of reproductive age more than the work burdens of other members of the household (Ferguson 1986). In three communities in Nepal, a study showed that deforestation has resulted in a significant increase in the time needed for women to collect fuelwood. In highland communities, the time needed to collect fuelwood increased from just over 1 hour per day to 2.5 hours per day (Kumar and Hotchkiss 1988). In areas of India where the forests have been ravaged, women and children must now trek 8–10 kilometres every day to get sufficient wood to cook the evening meal. Seven or eight years ago, a short walk of 1 or 2 kilometres was required (APDC 1990). In the Jayawijaya District, Irian Jaya Province, Indonesia, people began to use the high slopes of hills as the amount of land suitable for cultivation decreased. This led to soil erosion. The soil became infertile and food production decreased. The ultimate result was the deterioration of the quality of life for all, but in particular, women and children.[13]

> The most serious health hazards in the Tongu area are environmental degradation and poverty that stem from the resultant deterioration and loss of sources of livelihood. Economic activity surrounding the harvesting of clams, a predominantly female activity, has completely disappeared.
>
> — Dzodzi Tsikata, Institute of Statistical, Social and Economic Research, University of Ghana, Legon, Ghana

Women who are largely responsible for fetching water for their families may have to walk extra distances in the search for safe water because of environmental degradation. "The increasing run-off of agricultural chemicals and organic waste into rivers as well as siltation resulting from deforestation, [is] seriously affect[ing] the availability of clean, safe water for rural women" (APDC 1992, p. 56).

Researchers in a project in Burkino Faso examined the impact of fuelwood shortages on women's agricultural practices and on family nutritional intakes (Rathgeber 1990b, p. 500) and found that

As women are forced to spend longer periods of time searching for firewood, they have less time for agriculture. This in turn leads to lower crop

---

[13] See Handali, S., "Gender and women's health issues in Jayawijaya District, Irian Jaya, Indonesia." Unpublished paper submitted to the 1994–95 TDR/IDRC competition.

yields and a reduced level of food for family consumption as well as a smaller surplus for sale in local markets. At the same time, women are cooking less frequently and serving their families cheap storebought foods or foods cooked several hours earlier and often stored under unhealthy and unsanitary conditions.

Women's double and triple burden

To understand women's occupational health, the combined burdens and hazards of the many roles of women, including paid work and family responsibilities must be appreciated (Timoteo and Llanos-Cuentas 1994). Unfortunately, little research has focused on the double work day: "The fact that [women] often combine domestic or family responsibilities with their paid work ha[s] also been insufficiently studied from a health perspective" (Messing 1991, p. 7).

Women who have responsibilities both in the home and in the formal work force are often said to be suffering from a "double burden" (Messing 1991; Acevedo 1994; Berr 1994). Breilh also coined the term "triple load" or "threefold burden" to refer to the triple responsibilities that women may have: that is, responsibility for reproduction, productive work in the formal work force, and domestic work (Breilh 1994).

Bearing and raising children, often at very short intervals, breastfeeding them, and, at the same time, continuing to perform energy-consuming work loads (Alilio 1994) is an onerous task for many women. Studies in Tanzania have shown that most women continue to carry out energy-consuming work, such as fetching firewood and fuel, farming, cooking and washing, and taking care of children, until their last days of pregnancy and that they often do so without adequate caloric intake (Mpanju 1992).

Women throughout the world maintain almost exclusive responsibility for childcare and housework, and they invariably receive little support from other family members, such as husbands (Chavkin 1984; Breilh 1994). There is also a lack of institutional support, such as childcare centres, nurseries, and other services, particularly for working-class mothers.

Women are responsible for care of the home and family, regardless of whether or not they participate in the labour market. This reality represents a double workload for many Chilean women.

— Jasna Stiepovick and Julia Ramírez, Department of Nursing, Universidad de Concepción, Chile

---

The double shift and double load of working both inside and outside the home creates considerable physical and mental stress (Berr 1994), and the roles commonly conflict. Household duties do not begin and end at set times. Rather, they dominate, in one way or another, the entire day. While working, women invariably are thinking of their home and making decisions that affect the household and their children.

Poor conditions in the household may negatively affect a woman's work in the formal sphere. Fatigue may lead to higher rates of absenteeism and to frustration and discontent, which may cause high rates of turnover (ILO 1994). Being overburdened by numerous responsibilities may cause cumulative detrimental health effects such as fatigue, stress, and diminished resistance to disease and chronic illness. The significant demands may lead to the deprivation of physiological necessities, such as sleep. Furthermore, "[a] body tired out from taking care of a baby or ill parent may be less able to resist a virus ... or to protect itself against the solvents in cleaning solutions" (Messing 1991, p. 12).

CHARACTERISTICS OF WOMEN'S WORK

Many characteristics of women's work activities may have adverse consequences for the health and well-being of women. The following characteristics are associated with the kinds of work that a large number of women in the developing world perform. These characteristics are not specific to women's jobs, but they are common to many women's jobs.

Long working hours and lack of leisure time

When all forms of women's work are considered, women in the developing world work longer hours per day than men (Jacobson 1993; Paolisso and Leslie 1995). Although there are differences from region to region, estimates vary from 16 to 20 hours per day in some areas (Commonwealth Secretariat 1990; Acevedo 1994; Handali, see footnote 13). In African countries, for example, women farmers regularly have to put in 16-hour days. In Burkina Faso, India, Kenya, Nepal, and Niger, fuelwood collection has been found to require 3–5 hours per day and involves traveling distances of 3–10 kilometres (Agarwal 1986). As an illustration of the time-consuming labour that women perform, a study carried out in Africa showed that where modern technology is not available it takes about 13 hours to pound enough maize to feed a family for between 4 and 5 days (Butler et al. 1987).

Women's responsibilities as health providers demand a great deal of time from women: "[w]hen a mother has a very sick child, she has no rest day and night" (Wyss and Nandjingar 1995, p. 142). According to Richters (1994, p. 41): "[a] baby sick with diarrhoea, vomiting and fretful with fever will require an enormous amount of time if oral rehydration fluid of sufficient quantity is to be coaxed into its mouth spoonful by spoonful," as will breast-feeding "completely on demand ... for 18 months or 2 years as recommended in primary health care programs in the developing world."

On the windswept plains of western India, the women of Gotarka regard the arduous routine of their lives to be as natural as the monsoon rain. While their husbands sip tea and debate politics, the women, like their mothers and grandmothers before them, nurse and teach their children, fetch wood for fuel, lug pails of water, clean house, tend livestock, sow the fields. And keep the teapot boiling. "Our days are so long," says Manju Jayantila Darji, a mother of three. "We start our work when the moon is in the sky and when we finish it is there again."

— Stackhouse (1995a, p. D1).

Women, therefore, have less leisure or discretionary time available than men, particularly during certain agricultural seasons (Holmboe-Ottesen et al. 1989; McGuire and Popkin 1989). Not only do women work long hours, they have little control over when they work at a particular task. "The timing of women's work in collecting water and fuelwood, preparing foods, feeding family members, bathing, caring and educating children, working in fields or factories is very much demand driven according to the daily needs of the household" (Paolisso and Leslie 1995, p. 60).

Such long working days often results in extreme fatigue. Lack of leisure time may also make it extremely difficult for women to find the opportunity to properly attend to a health problem (Berr 1994).

Poorly paid or unpaid

Sufficient wages are essential for health: "without assuring adequate wages, it is meaningless to discuss health or other measures to ensure health" (Misch 1992, p. 24). Sufficient wages are necessary to afford nutritious and adequate food, proper accommodations with healthier sources of water and environmentally safe power, as well as education. According to Messing (1991, p. 10): "a too-low income can ... worsen health by diminishing access to adequate nutrition and housing and by increasing stress levels."

However, much of women's work is underpaid and undervalued. The average salary received by women is always lower than that of their male counterparts (UN 1991; Acevedo 1994). Worldwide, female wages are, on average, only two-thirds those of men. In parts of Africa and Asia, the wage gap in male–female earnings reaches 50% (UNDIESA 1991). Furthermore, women perform essential household roles that are not considered to be economically important and are not paid.

The observations of Gerelsuren and Erdenechimeg (1995), of the Mongolian Women's Federation, are all too familiar:

> Although Mongolian law enshrines the principle of equal pay for work of equal value, women on average receive lower wages than men. This is related to the fact that women occupy most of the lower-paying and nonprofessional jobs. Although the government has issued some resolutions about flexible working hours for women, improved labour safety, and the creation of healthy working conditions for women, women continue to work in unhealthy environments.

Job segregation and discrimination contributes to wage differentials between women and men (ILO 1985). Women tend to work in jobs with little prestige and status (UN 1991; Acevedo 1994). Furthermore, even when women do the same work as men and have the same educational qualifications, women typically receive less pay than men. The feminization of occupations traditionally carried out by men tends to devaluate them (Acevedo 1994).

Women's perceived role as secondary breadwinners is another major reason cited to explain unequal pay between the sexes for the same work (Grandea 1994).

The salaries [at the textile factory] were not sufficient to meet basic needs. The entire month's salary was needed simply to purchase and prepare food.

— Joseph Carasco, Centre for Basic Research, Kampala, Uganda

Low-waged working women are more likely to suffer from a lack of nutritional energy, anemia, and high stress levels (Carasco 1994). Because women tend to use a high proportion of whatever income they do earn to meet family nutrition and basic amenity needs, low-wages translate into little or no remaining income for women to use for their own health needs (Paolisso and Leslie 1995).

Poor working women, with insufficient time to earn, care for their families, and conscientiously look after their health, are also unlikely to take

The base salaries of workers must be raised to provide for a good standard of living if higher occupational health and safety standards are to be achieved. The Labour Resources Centre has found that the most important concern for workers is wages. Workers will even carry out hazardous jobs or use hazardous chemicals if they are paid an allowance for the job.

— Josie Zaini, Education and Research Association for Consumers, Subong Jaya, Malaysia (see Labour Resources Centre 1995)

time away from work to use health services: "sick leave may be unavailable or too costly for women with low incomes, [and] they may be forced to neglect their own health needs" (Messing 1991, p. 10).

Economic crisis further compounds health problems for women with low incomes. "When food prices rise and wages fall, a woman must spend more time finding ways to satisfy her family's hunger, travelling further to cheaper shops or markets, preparing cheaper food, and often eating less herself in order to feed her husband and children" (Vickers, 1991, p. 15).

There may also be a link between income levels and safety in the workplace. When incomes for women in a society are higher, and greater employment possibilities are available, women may have some degree of choice about whether or not they continue to work in a situation that poses hazards to their health and safety. In societies that offer fewer opportunities to women, the only choice available may be between a low-paying job with little or no occupational health and safety protection and no job at all.

If working wages are insufficient to meet basic needs, women may be forced to look for income from other sources. The extent to which women engage in secondary employment and the effects of this employment on health effects need more attention. Women with limited resources may also engage in prostitution to generate additional income (Standing and Kisekka 1989; Pauw 1993; Strebel 1994). According to the WHO (1994a, p. 59), "in hard times, some [women] find it necessary to trade sex for money, food, or shelter." Multiple sexual partnerships, without condom use, leads to an increased risk of STDs, including AIDS.

Female-headed households

It is impossible to discuss women and their working environment without considering the fact that many women are the sole or primary source of family income. The increasing number of single women who have children and are heads of households worldwide is a result of a number of factors: national and international migration of men in the search for work; divorce; widow-hood; wars; desertion; and the increasing number of births to unpartnered adolescent women. It is estimated that female-headed households make up one-quarter of households around the world (UN 1995). In the Caribbean, women constitute up to 35% of all heads of households; in parts of sub-Saharan Africa, the figure is 40–45% (UN 1995).

Female-headed households are particularly disadvantaged and eco-nomically vulnerable. As a result of the lack of educational opportunities that many women face and the difficulties of obtaining well-paid secure employment, a smaller amount of money often comes into the female-headed households than into male-headed households. In Canada, single-parent families headed by women are on the rise and most of them (57.2% in 1992) live in poverty (Status of Women Canada 1994). As stated by Richters (1994):

> Women appear to be the only financial support for as many as a third of the world's families. Because such mothers are often poorly educated, without investment capital, and attempt to do two jobs at once (domes-tic and wage work), female-headed households tend to be poor.

In female-headed households, coping with limited living space and scarce resources has a high cost on the physical and mental health of these women (Acevedo 1994). The deterioration of public services particularly affects these women.

The transformation of subsistence-agricultural economies into income-generation economies may lead to an increased number of female-headed household and have negative impacts on health. Herrera and Lobo-Guerrera (1994) explained that some indigenous women in the Orinoco and Amazon basins faced significantly increased workloads when their husbands left the household for many months of the year in search of income-generation activities. Although the women had their agricultural produce from the *conuco* (small plot of land), they did not have the protein foods, such as meat and fish, that their husbands usually obtained.

Therefore, as stressed by Leslie (1992, p. 15),

> Given the increasing prevalence of female-headed households, and dif-ferential findings in terms of the welfare of women and children living in female-headed households, local social science research is urgently needed to investigate factors that compound or mitigate poverty and poor health within such households.

Low positions

Throughout the world, women's subordinate position in society is reflected in the dearth of women in positions that involve the supervision and direction of others. In the majority of countries around the world, women hold only a small proportion (between 10 and 30%) of management positions, and even fewer (less than 5%) of the very highest posts (ILO 1993). In addition, women are poorly represented in the ranks of power, policy, and decision-making. Indeed, women make up less than 5% of the world's heads of state, the heads of major corporations, and the top positions in international organizations (UN 1991).

Unemployment

In many developing countries, unemployment for females is much higher than for males. Women are particularly vulnerable to fluctuating economic conditions because they are least likely to benefit for job expansion and the first to suffer from job contraction. Unemployment, especially for poorer people, is associated with deteriorating physical and mental health.

In the English-speaking Caribbean, for example, women and young adults (under 25 years of age) are the most vulnerable groups in the labour force, and women are particularly disadvantaged. Of the 191 000 unemployed persons in Jamaica in 1989, 57.2% were 25 years old or younger, but 64.5% of the unemployed were women (Planning Institute of Jamaica 1989). In 1991, the unemployment rate for females in Jamaica (23.1%) was more than twice that for males (9.3%) (ILO 1994). Similar patterns were reported for Guyana in 1986 and Trinidad in 1988 (PAHO and WHO 1992).

Women are less likely to show up in unemployment statistics because they are more likely to be involved in temporary part-time jobs and the informal work force.

— Doris Acevedo, Carabodo University, Maracay, Venezuela

Women may not look for work because there is no work suitable to them or they have become discouraged because they are victims of prejudice and discrimination (Nuss 1989). In addition to general discrimination on the basis of sex, women may experience discrimination if they do not measure up to a certain notion of feminine beauty (Acevedo 1994). Managers may hire or promote women on the basis of their attractiveness (Humphrey 1987). In Venezuela, for example, advertisements for secretaries and receptionists often require a "good appearance," an attribute that is not demanded of men (Acevedo 1994).

Part-time and voluntary work

Women are more likely to be part-time workers than men, in part because women try to fit their work around family responsibilities. Activities such as market trading and street vending offer this kind of flexibility. In West Africa, women dominate this type of work; for example, they make up 93% of the market traders in Accra, 87% in Lagos, and 60% in Dakar. However, significant portions of the world's women are engaged in involuntary temporary, part-time, or seasonal work. Part-time workers, usually excluded from trade-union membership, have no channels for negotiating better terms for work (Grandea 1994).

Voluntary social work is usually done by women, with little recognition and no remuneration. For example, women comprise most of the volunteers in hospitals, self-help clinics, and other community organizations. In Latin America, women have formed networks such as housewives associations and mothers' clubs to help them to meet their basic daily needs (Jacquette 1986). For example, in the settlements around the larger cities of Peru, many women have created and are running "Mothers' clubs" and "Milk glass committees," which are organizations aimed at providing effective relief from deteriorating economic and health conditions (Timoteo and Llanos-Cuentas 1994).

Women's lives, and women's workloads, are hit the hardest by economic crisis and adjustment policies because women must take on even greater responsibilities. Reductions in health, child-care, and education services mean that women are forced to provide, on a private or individual basis, social services that were formerly provided by the state (Commonwealth Secretariat 1990; Vickers 1991; Acevedo 1994).

Shift work

Shift work, which has become increasingly prevalent in the industrial sector as automated equipment is introduced, may lead to gastrointestinal disorders, nervous disorders, and sleep disturbances (such as fatigue, light sleep, and insomnia). Anxiety, confusion, irritability, nervousness, depression, and concentration difficulties have been linked to shift work (Labour Resource Centre 1995).

The conditions surrounding shift work, which often involves night work, may also decrease the amount of time that a woman has with her family in the home. For example, Haile (1994) reported that women night workers in Ethiopia are often forced to sleep in the factory after work because there is a lack of adequate transportation services to their homes. If a woman takes a service bus that lets her off at a central point, she will be exposed to the risk of both rape and robbery. Therefore, many women decide to spend the night at the work area and often get insufficient sleep.

Laws are of no consequence if the machinery of enforcement and other administrative mechanisms are weak and if those who are meant to be protected by laws are unaware of their existence.

— Josie Zaini, Education and Research Association for Consumers, Subong Jaya, Malaysia (see Labour Resource Centre 1995)

Lack of occupational health and safety protection

Occupational health and safety standards and enforcement measures are necessary to ensure the promotion and maintenance of the highest degree of physical, mental, and social well-being of workers in all occupations (Puta 1994). To ensure the health and safety of workers, measures must be taken to establish and maintain a safe and healthy working environment and to prevent illness and injury related to working conditions.

Women often work in unregulated industries that may be outside the scope of occupational health and safety legislation (ILO 1985; World Bank 1993). In situations in which legislation is in place, it may not be enforced, which renders it useless.

The devastating implications of the absence of enforced safety standards were realized in Bangkok, Thailand, in May 1993, when a lack of fire-safety precautions led to the death of over 200 employees and to severe injuries to hundreds more, when a toy factory burned to the ground. Most of the victims were young Thai women who earned the equivalent of US $6 a day stuffing toy dolls. Fire alarms were not functioning and there were no smoke detectors, fire escapes, or fire drills. Because some exits were routinely locked shut, hundreds of workers were forced to jump from the third and fourth stories in an attempt to escape. The factory was owned by interests from Hong Kong, Taiwan, and Thailand and produced dolls for multinational toy companies in the United States.

According to Kittipak Thavisri, a labour specialist at Thammasat University in Bangkok (IHT 1993, p. 15),

> Public safety is costly ... to attract foreign investors .... You have to overlook some of the labor regulations .... Much the same situation prevails in

> Many workers, particularly women, work in jobs that are not
> protected by labour and social security legislation or work under
> noncontractual conditions. [A significant number] of noncontractual
> female workers [in Chile] work in agriculture, domestic services,
> fisheries, and commerce industries.
>
> — Ximena Díaz Berr, Salaried Women in Industry and Fruitculture, Santiago, Chile

thousand of other factories in Thailand .... Insufficient attention is paid in Asia to safe working conditions in an economic climate where the stress of manufacturers is often on keeping production costs as low as possible.

In fact, throughout Southeast Asia, labour safety laws have not kept pace with economic development. In some nations, there are no laws at all. In others that do have laws, there is practically no enforcement (Shenom 1993, p. 3).

Greater steps must be taken to ensure that adequate occupational health and safety standards, and enforcement measures, are put into place with regard to the risks associated with women's work.

In industrialized countries, attention to women's occupational safety has usually focused on safeguarding their reproductive capacity by protecting them from work environments deemed dangerous to fertility (Eines 1993) and on protecting the health of the fetus. The fact that reproductive damage may also be experienced by men has been largely neglected until recently.

Women must also be on guard for the possibility that protective legislation may be used against them. For example, protective legislation has been used to justify discriminatory labour practices and policies to keep women out of better paid jobs held mostly by men. In an American legal case, for example, the Supreme Court of the United States found that protective legislation excluding "women who are pregnant or who are capable

> Although there are a number of International Labour Organisation
> conventions that specifically address the protection of the health
> of women workers, their implementation by member countries has
> been less than desired.
>
> — Fekerte Haile, International Labour Organisation, Addis Ababa, Ethiopia

of bearing children," was used to prevent women from obtaining high-paying jobs (Johnson Controls 1991, p. 1198).

Other types of legislation aimed at protecting women may also end up depressing their wages or discouraging their employment. For example, many countries have legislation that establishes standard periods of maternity leave and other special benefits for women. Such legislation usually requires employers to provide these benefits to female workers, effectively increasing the cost of hiring them. To avoid paying maternity benefits, some garment manufacturers in Bangledesh hire young women only on a daily or casual basis (World Bank 1995). Acevedo (1994) reported that, in Venezuela, changes to the employment law intended to benefit women[14] have actually served to hurt some women. In response to the legislation, some employers in the industrial sector are actively recruiting only women who are beyond childbearing age or are replacing female employees with men. Some companies, before they hire a woman of childbearing age, are even demanding that women produce medical certificates attesting to their sterilization (Acevedo 1994).

Lack of union support

Women may suffer additional work stress in situations where they have no protective associations to support them when necessary. For example, workers in some export-producing free-trade zones, such as in Sri Lanka, are not permitted by law to form unions (APDC 1990).

Where unions do exist, they are often underrepresented by women. The Labour Resource Centre (1995) reported that, in Malaysia, legislation requires that a safety committee must be established in places of employment with more than 40 employees. Although the legislation specifies the number of employees and employers that must be on the committee, it does not specify representation on the basis of sex.

The trade-union leadership was dominated by male workers who are not usually sensitive to gender issues. As a result, female workers had less recourse to an organized group that was supposed to be there for the assistance of all employees.

— Joseph Carasco, Centre for Basic Research, Kampala, Uganda

---

[14] Such as lengthening the time for pregnancy leave from 12 to 16 weeks and prohibiting job dismissal during the year following the birth of a child.

Interests of female workers — such as childcare, sexual harrassment, lack of access to capital, social subordination, and health and safety issues — are rarely the interests of traditional trade unions. In a study of male-dominated trade unions in female-dominated occupations (Rathgeber 1990a, p. 16), researchers found that

> Women's concerns were usually not articulated by male trade union representatives ... but women themselves were reluctant to become involved in union activities because they felt that they lacked the necessary verbal skills or they were unable to combine time-consuming union activism with their domestic responsibilities .... Even when women have achieved high level qualifications or have become members of trade unions which supposedly protect their interests, gender still operates as a powerful intervening variable in the context of actual workplace experiences.

Strategies need to be developed to increase the representation of women in trade unions and to make trade unions more responsive to the needs of their membership, including females.

Lack of contracts

Many women in developing countries work in situations without contracts and therefore receive no health coverage or social security protection (Machado 1993; Berr 1994). Employers are also absolved from giving non-contractual workers, or temporary contract workers, maternity leave or rights to use company health clinics. For example, Zaini (unpublished)[15] explained that, because a pregnant woman working for a contractor on a Malaysian plantation is not entitled to paid maternity leave, "[she] will be back in the plantation a week after her delivery for her income is vital to the family's survival."

A study of 300 women who pick grapes for export in Chile[16] revealed that 65% of the women worked with a taskwork contract and another 14.3% worked without any contract (Medel and Riquelme 1992). In the best of cases, some of these women were protected against accidents and work-related diseases during the months in which they were employed. However, if the women later experienced health problems related to their hard work during the fruit-picking season, protection was not provided (Berr 1994).

Women are often involved in temporary or part-time work, and they are usually not eligible for insurance against accidents or disease, even if they have contracts. Women working in agriculture, as domestic servants, and in

---

[15] See Zaini, J., "Women in Malaysian plantations: health and medicines." Cited in APDC (1990).

[16] Grape picking is one of the most important sources of female employment within Chile's productive sector.

fisheries and fruit picking, often work in noncontractual relationships (Berr 1994). In Brazil, approximately one-third of the 15 million women who made up with female work force in 1985 were employed as domestic workers. These women, who usually earn below minimum wage, often do not have employment contracts and are not covered by the social welfare system, which provides such benefits as health insurance, pension, and retirement benefits (ILO 1985; Machado 1993). The percentage of women without contracts is highest among low-income groups and rural women.

There has been an increase in the use of homeworkers in many parts of the world to reduce labour costs. Companies that use homeworkers usually have a long subcontracting chain. The last and most precarious link is the work performed predominantly by women in their homes. These women have no formal work contracts, no social security, and no coverage against accidents and diseases (Berr 1994). If a homeworker is ill, she cannot take medical leave. In the case of injury or illness during work, the cost of medical treatment is borne by the worker or their families. It is not the responsibility of the employer (Prompunthum and Kerdpol 1985; ILO 1992b).

Lack of information on health and safety risks

Women often lack information on the extent to which detrimental working conditions can lead to negative health effects. For example, women may be unaware of the toxic effects of chemical materials that they handle. Although this may sometimes be because information is unavailable, in other cases, it is because they have not been properly informed of the hazards. LaDou (1993) reported that lack of knowledge about the dangers of pesticides is pervasive among workers, employers, and even pesticide sellers. Workers — and all others who are in contact with harmful agents — have a right to know about suspected hazards, and training programs should be instituted.

The Labour Resource Centre (1995) pointed out, however, that it is a constant struggle to educate workers about health and safety concerns. Many workers, primarily concerned with having work and receiving better wages,

---

Most workers, especially in developing countries, are unaware of the toxic effects of the chemical materials they handle. Occupational health and safety education programs should be provided to all workers.

— Anne Kamoto Puta, Zambian Organization of Occupational Health and Safety, Ndola, Zambia

Health is not viewed as a priority area, compared with urgent issues such as salaries [and] stability of employment. Women are often unaware of the relationship between working conditions and the deterioration of their health.

— Ximena Díaz Berr, Salaried Women in Industry and Fruitculture, Santiago, Chile

do not consider workplace health and safety issues to be a priority. Indeed, some workers may even agree to carry out hazardous jobs or use hazardous chemicals if they are paid an extra allowance for the job.

Sexual harassment

There is a growing recognition of the extent to which women may be subjected to sexual harassment on the job (Ahikirie 1991). Employers may demand sex in return for access to, or continuance in, a job, promotions, or salary increases. A woman who desperately needs the work may find herself unable to refuse the demands for sexual favours. A woman who is subjected to sexual harassment may suffer mental and psychological damage as well as adverse physiological reactions, such as gastritis and dizziness (Acevedo 1994).

As described by Humphrey (1987, p. 140),

> They [women] can be sacked by foremen and managers for rejecting advances, sacked if a relationship comes to an end, and in many cases sacked if they denounce the offender .... Possibly more pervasive and generalized are the public humiliations and demeaning of women through bullying, shouting, abuse and disciplinary warnings ... such practices seemed quite common in Brazilian factories.

Stress

Increased attention is being given to the extent to which stress affects the health and well-being of individuals. There are a number of psychosocial factors found in the workplace that are related to stress levels: the number of hours worked; the level of job satisfaction; the complexity of tasks; the degree of supervision; and the organizational structure. Stress can by provoked by other workplace conditions such as noise, chemicals, and sexual harassment (Messing 1991). Stress has also been linked with few rest periods, constant demands, inability to talk with co-workers, and repetitive work (Messing 1991).

Stress is an important hazard associated with work for many women. The competing demands on women from their work and family can be a significant source of stress in both developing and industrialized countries. Several studies in industrialized countries have demonstrated that the stress associated with balancing paid work outside the home with childrearing and household management responsibilities can lead to decreased productivity, tardiness, absenteeism, turnover, poor morale, reduced life satisfaction, and poorer mental health (Lee et al. 1994). Furthermore, women often have higher levels of stress than men because of the social conditions under which they live, conditions of economic inequality, poverty, and marginality.

> *The blurring of work and home boundaries, more pronounced for women, can lead to high stress levels. Working women who are also trying to cope with responsibilities in the home may suffer from migraines, nervousness, and depression.*
>
> — Ng Yen Yen, Senator to the Malaysian Parliament, Pahang, Malaysia

In some industries that predominantly employ females, the fast pace of the work regime and the domination of women's lives by production targets may lead to a chronic state of ill-health. Workers, under the constant threat of dismissal if quotas are not met, may experience headaches, fatigue, stomach ulcers, constant colds, sleeping problems, high blood pressure, and palpations of the heart (APDC 1990). However, there have been few systematic studies of stress in female-dominated industries.

Some research has been conducted in Latin America on stress among women in the paid work force. Berr (1994) reported results from a study conducted by the Centre for Women's Studies in Chile on risk factors associated with stress among females who work in the fruit and garment industries. A stress index was developed based on the presence of three stress-related diseases (neurosis, ulcers, and gastritis) reported by working women. This was followed by an analysis of factors associated with the stress index. From these control values (women who have never suffered from any of the three diseases), an analysis was undertaken to identify risk factors associated with stress.

In the garment industry, women who reported that they suffered from stress-related illnesses were 3.7 times more likely to be economically responsible for the household; 2.0 times more likely to be exposed to environmental noise; and 2.8 times more likely to have suffered some type of accident at the workplace. In the case of female fruit pickers, women were more likely to suffer from a stress-related illness if they devoted more than 2 hours a day to household work (8.5 times more); feared dismissal (3.5 times more); and worked in a forced physical position (2.1 times more). In packing plants, stressful working conditions were related to the rigorousness of the work and the long working hours. Women working in packing plants were more susceptible to stress when they feared dismissal (3.4 times more) and worked in a noisy environment (3.9 times more).

Breilh (1994) presented survey results with regard to stress among women in the civil service in Ecuador. A high proportion of the women surveyed were in a state of stress. He reported that high stress levels among female civil servants were associated with repetitive and dull work, poor organization, and too much work. It was also shown that women who stood a great deal during their work were most affected by stress.

High stress levels were also linked to lack of support with domestic responsibilities. Over 50% of the working women surveyed by Breilh (1994) carried out a large amount of domestic work with no support of any kind. Among the workers with a husband or partner, a very small percentage reported that they received help in the home from their partners. Only 10% of partners helped out with domestic labour, and 27% of the men participated in tasks involving family care and attention.

Breilh reported that there was a significant decrease of severe stress in workers with the highest levels of recreation. However, because of cultural restrictions and lack of time, recreation time for female workers was minimal, and the full protective effect of recreation was therefore not realized. Women invariably have little time for themselves, for personal projects, leisure, or recreational activities.

Breilh also established a relationship between a stressful working environment and the presence of a menstruation disturbance. The percentage of women with polymenorrhea (increased menstruation) almost tripled in workers with a high level of stress. Women who were experiencing high stress levels were also found to be most likely to suffer from other ailments, such as intercurrent infections. Psychological stress can also result in amenorrhea among women (RCNRT 1993).

Possible detrimental effects on reproduction

Women's work activities may also lead to reproductive difficulties. Heavy loads, for example, may lead to a prolapsed uterus and are associated with menstrual disorders, miscarriage, and stillbirth (NCSEW 1988). A study in Maharashtna, India, which addressed heavy agricultural work, found that there was a high incidence of stillbirths and premature births during the peak season for rice cultivation season when everyone, including women whose pregnancy is almost full-term, are in the fields the whole day. "The work involves squatting and bending for hours. Such physical strain and pressure in the uterus can lead to premature labour as well as births" (Batliwala 1988, p. 33).

Other potential reproductive problems for farm women may include the following (Engberg 1993, p. 873):

✦ Disruption of the menstrual cycle;

✦ Infertility;

✦ Fetal malformation;

✦ Cancer among offspring;

✦ Growth retardation; and

✦ Abnormal postnatal development of infants because of chemicals passed to breastmilk.

Certain working conditions, such as shift work, irregular schedules, and temperature variations, may change the menstrual cycle of a woman (Acevedo 1994). Some studies have shown that cold, exposure to solvents, or lifting weights at a fast pace can produce menstrual pain (dysmenorrhoea) (Messing 1991).

Prolonged standing, shift work, long working days, radiation, and exposure to certain chemicals may contribute to the number of spontaneous abortions among working women (Patrick 1991, cited in Koblinsky, Timyan et al. 1993; Acevedo 1994). Borges (1993) noted that high-stress jobs, and low task control, increased the risk that a woman would experience a premature birth (Acevedo 1994).

A study carried out in La Victoria, Venezuela, assessed the health status of a group of female textile workers and compared them with women from the same neighbourhood who did not work outside the home (Borges and Acevedo 1994). Generally, the textile workers tended to have poorer living conditions and lower levels of schooling and to be significantly more likely to be the financial head of the household than the women who did not work outside the home. The textile workers also had significantly more spontaneous abortions and significantly lower birthweights of their newborns than women who worked exclusively in the home.[17] The characteristics of work in the textile factory, including long working hours at an assembly line, the intense working pace, and prolonged standing, combined with poor living conditions and the burden of caring for a family, may have contributed to these reproductive difficulties.

---

[17] See Borges, A.; Acevedo, D. Salud reproductiva en textileras y amas de casa, La Victoria, Aragua, Venezuela. Unpublished.

Positive aspects of women's work

Work may also have many positive health benefits for women. In industrialized countries, evidence suggests that, at least for women who have a positive attitude toward work, there is a strong positive association between women's employment and women's health (Repetti et al. 1989; Rodin and Ickovics 1990). As well, it appears that the mental and physical health of employed women is significantly better than the health of women who stay at home (McDaniel 1987).

Women working in the formal work force may experience heightened self-esteem and confidence in their abilities and decisions. The workplace environment also offers the opportunity to obtain social support from co-workers (Leslie 1992; Debert-Ribeiro 1993). Juggling multiple roles (such as in the household and in the paid work force) can result in higher self-esteem and greater happiness and may act as a shield against depression (Ayers et al. 1993). Employment's protective effect has been found to be greater for women who hold professional and managerial positions than for those in blue-collar occupations (Hazuda et al. 1986).

Because working conditions in developing countries are quite different from industrialized countries, it is difficult to generalize from data obtained in industrialized countries. It is therefore important that the health consequences of women's increased participation in the work force of developing countries be systematically and fully explored.

Chapter 6

Tropical Disease

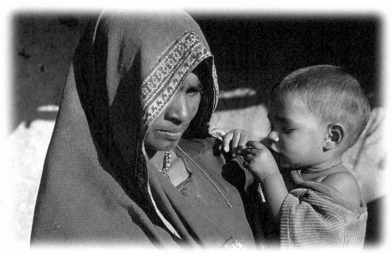

> *For the most part, the literature assumes that the effects of tropical diseases on men and women are similar, with the proviso that women will suffer more acutely during pregnancy and childbearing. While it may be accurate, the research does not go far enough in analyzing the adverse effects of tropical diseases on women within the context of their multiple economic, social, cultural, and private roles.*
>
> — Rathgeber and Vlassoff (1993, p. 513)

The tropical diseases[18] are among the most pervasive and neglected diseases of the world. Malarial parasites, for example, are found in approximately 100 countries, and annually infect an estimated 270 million people, kill up to 2 million more (far more than does AIDS), and cause at least 100 million cases of acute illness (Cowley 1992; WHO 1993). Approximately 200 million people are infected with schistosomiasis in 76 countries, and about 200 000 die each year from the disease (WHO 1991). It is estimated that there are over 12 million leishmaniasis cases worldwide and approximately 350 million people are considered at risk (WHO 1990). About 20 million people are affected by onchocerciasis (Stephenson 1987; Warren et al. 1993), and it is estimated that 10–12 million people suffer from leprosy infection (Htoon et al. 1993).

The gender dimensions of tropical diseases have been largely neglected. The area has traditionally been dominated by a biomedical perspective, and the subjects of research have tended to be men and children. When the effects of tropical diseases on women have been addressed, research has "focused primarily on sex differences, particularly related to pregnancy and reproduction, and has not examined these in relation to broader social roles and responsibilities" (Rathgeber and Vlassoff 1993, p. 513).

Although a biomedical viewpoint has predominated, there remain many outstanding questions about the influence of biological factors on tropical diseases, including the effect of sex on the susceptibility and intensity of infection and progression of disease (Brabin and Brabin 1992; Duncan 1992;

The authors thank Lori Jones Arsenault of IDRC, a collaborating author on this chapter, for her valuable contribution.

[18] Including malaria, schistosomiasis, filariasis (lymphatic filariasis and onchocerciasis), trypanosomiasis (Chagas' disease and African trypanosomiasis), leprosy, cholera, and leishmaniasis.

Michelson 1992; Vlassoff 1994). Women appear to "mount a better immune response" to some tropical diseases (such as malaria, leprosy, and visceral leishmaniasis) and "either have a stronger natural immunity or a stronger and more rapid cellular response" (Agyepong 1992, p. 179). However, many researchers have been quick to point out that any advantage gained by sex hormones in women may be quickly lost during pregnancy when the immune system becomes depressed and susceptibility to disease increases (Brabin and Brabin 1992). In the developing world, many cycles of pregnancy and lactation, often beginning at an early age, heighten women's vulnerability to disease. Parasitic infection in pregnancy can lead to malnutrition and deterioration in women's disease state and also have serious implications for fetal growth and development (Brabin and Brabin 1992).

The depressed health of women, which in Africa is related to general malnutrition and infection and complications of pregnancy and childbirth, is one of the reasons for the high levels of mortality and morbidity in women from malaria. Nutritional anemia ... contribute[s] considerably to the recurrence of episodes of malaria. In one study conducted in Nzega, in central Tanzania, anemia and clinical malaria during pregnancy were identified in 87% of 1 072 women surveyed.

— Martin Sarikiaeli Alilio, National Institute for Medical Research, Muheza Tanga, Tanzania

Intercurrent infections and poor nutrition, other factors that compromise women's immunological reactivity, may further modulate this response (Ulrich et al. 1992). As a result of discriminatory feeding practices and female poverty, girls and women suffer disproportionately from poor nutrition and are impaired in their ability to fight disease (Duncan 1992). The depressed health status of women also influences their disease recovery.

There is also a growing body of research that suggests that "morbidity and mortality rates reflect not so much sex differences in the biology of disease, but the mediation of disease through cultural and social circumstances" (Manderson 1994, p. 1; see also Tandon 1995). The sociocultural dimensions of tropical diseases include the ways in which gender affects the transmission of disease and risk of infection, the recognition of, and response to, signs of infection, the social experience of illness, access to care, and the effectiveness of interventions.

GENDER-DIFFERENTIATED
"LIFE SPACES"

An understanding of the patterned use and management of "local life spaces" by men and women is central to understanding why women face different levels of exposure to infection than men and why the risk of infection to some tropical diseases varies from one geographic area to another (Parker 1992; Kettel 1996). For example, although women and men, overall, appear to be equally affected by schistosomiasis and malaria, male to female ratios of disease prevalence vary considerably from region to region depending on the sexual division of labour and responsibility (Anyangwe et al. 1994; Vlassoff and Bonilla 1994). "In this respect, there is no clear direction of sex bias: in some instances it is men who carry the burden of infection, in other instances, women" (Manderson 1994, p. 2).

Women play a key role in food production in many parts of the developing world, and their agricultural responsibilities, which include planting, weeding, harvesting, threshing, and winnowing, can expose them to an increased risk of tropical diseases such as malaria and onchocerciasis. Malarial parasites are transmitted to humans through the bite of specific vectors of *Anopheles* mosquitos (Nájera et al. 1993). Onchocerciasis is caused by the parasitic worm *Onchocerca volvulus* and is spread through the bite of blackflies that transmit worm larvae from infected to uninfected people. In parts of Nigeria, women spend more time in high transmission zones than men, and are more exposed to the bites of disease vectors for onchocerciasis and malaria (Amazigo 1994).

Despite women's important participation in agricultural activities, sometimes their activities are not fully acknowledged and the risks associated with their work are not thoroughly identified by researchers. For example,

Women and men lead gender-differentiated lives, and ... in many communities ... women and men do not inhabit the same "life spaces." They may live in the same city or village, they may work on the same farm, they may sleep in the same room in the same household, but from the time they rise, until the time they go to bed, they may actually occupy and use very different life spaces, and they may be exposed to very different environmental illnesses as a result.

— Kettel (1995)

> There are close links between women's gender roles and their
> susceptibility to chronic or recurrent ill health from urinary
> schistosomiasis and malaria.
>
> — Stella Anyangwe, Faculty of Medicine and Biomedical Sciences, University of
> Yaoundé I, Yaoundé, Cameroon

Amazigo (1994) noted that, in the assessment of exposure to onchocerciasis vector bites, the tasks predominantly carried out by women were often ignored. If the full range of women's activities are not considered in estimates of disease prevalence, the extent of female infection can be underestimated (Vlassoff and Bonilla 1994).

When both women and men perform farm work, their different responsibilities can create disparate risks. In Simbok, Cameroon, men specialized in cash-crop activities; whereas, women were primarily responsible for tending food crops, such as groundnut and maize (Anyangwe et al. 1994). Women usually undertook the weeding and harvesting of their food crops before dawn so that they could be at the markets by daybreak. Predawn is one of the peak periods for the transmission of malaria and the timing of their activities meant that women were at greater risk for this disease (Anyangwe et al. 1994). Although most women wore trousers to farm, their arms and faces were rarely protected.

Laundry and fetching water are predominantly female chores. Because mosquito habitats and malaria transmission sites are focused around water, women's regular visits to springs or rivers infested with mosquito larvae can increase their risk of malaria (Nájera et al. 1993; Anyangwe et al. 1994).

Although some sociocultural factors can predispose women to malaria infection, other practices can safeguard females. Cultural restrictions on women's mode of dress or on their freedom of movement may protect them from mosquito bites (Silva 1988). Spending the early evening hours in the kitchen where smoke from fires protects them from mosquitos will offer women further protection (while exposing them to air pollution). If men, on the other hand, spend significant amounts of time sitting outside in the evening or sleep outdoors, they will be exposed to an increased risk of malaria in endemic regions (Reubin 1992).

Schistosomiasis is the broad descriptive term given to a group of helminth (worm) infections caused by schistosomes. The majority of human infections are caused by four related species that develop within an aquatic snail host and are transmitted to humans through direct skin penetration or the drinking of contaminated water. Transmission of water-borne diseases, such as schistosomiasis, is linked to culturally prescribed and gender-differentiated responsibilities and activities. Women tend to have more frequent and intense water contacts than men because they are usually responsible for gathering water and washing clothes (Parker 1992). Infection rates for women vary from region to region depending on the time of day these activities take place (which, in turn, impacts on the degree of cercarial contact) (Michelson 1992).

In Kotto Barombi, Cameroon, schistosomiasis posed a particular risk for women and girls who were responsible for water collection, laundry, bathing children, washing utensils, lake-side fishing, and wetland-rice cultivation (Anyangwe et al. 1994). Each of these activities required constant and prolonged contact with the infested lakes; in fact, women sometimes spent as much as 6–10 hours at a time in the lake waist deep, urinating and defecating when necessary (Michelson 1992; Anyangwe et al. 1994). Female children were exposed to the water as early as 3 years of age. Women's water-contact activities were often very social — groups of women carried out their work together and mundane tasks were transformed into times for social entertainment and information sharing. Given the enjoyable nature of the activities, women rejected interventions aimed at reducing their contact with the lake. In comparison with women, men had little direct exposure to the water. Their fishing activities were conducted from canoes in the middle of the lake.

In other societies, however, cultural dictates may result in men having significant contact with infected waters. In communities where males swim and bathe for recreation in reservoirs, canals, and rivers or fish, men and boys may be more exposed to water-borne diseases than women (Michelson

---

Utensils and clothes are washed on the shores of the lake, where water is also fetched for household cleaning, cooking, and sometimes bathing. Basket-fishing is a female occupation. Women wade a few metres into the lake and position their fishing baskets under rocks from where they catch small fish and shrimps. Females in Kotto are, by virtue of the traditional and culturally prescribed gender roles and water-contact patterns, exposed to urinary schistosomiasis, which they help propagate by promiscuous urinating and defecating in the lake.

— Stella Anyangwe, Faculty of Medicine and Biomedical Sciences, University of Yaoundé I, Yaoundé, Cameroon

1992). Infection rates for schistosomiasis can be significantly lower for women in Muslim regions of the world because of restrictions on women's activities (Amazigo 1994; Anyangwe et al. 1994). In Muslim societies, women often remain secluded in their households, and men are responsible for almost all activities that are linked to the possibility of contamination from water, such as obtaining water for cooking and washing. Religious practices involving water contact, such as ablution and *wadu* (ritual washing), are also strictly male activities. Higher prevalence rates of schistosomiasis can occur among men in Muslim communities when ablution pools at Mosques become contaminated with host snails and serve as transmission sites (Michelson 1992).

Males are generally at a greater risk than females for leishmaniasis, a group of sandfly-transmitted parasitic diseases, and this risk has traditionally been associated with their occupations (Ayele 1988; Nandy et al. 1988). Activities that most typically place men at risk throughout endemic areas include deforestation, agriculture, hunting, road construction, and work on water-resource development projects. In Peru, leishmaniasis is associated with the opening of new roads, oil extraction, lumbering, and gold mining (Timotea and Llanos-Cuentas 1994). Differences in clothing patterns, with women being better clothed than men, may also expose men more than women (Thakur 1981). Although women are usually less exposed to the bite of leishmaniasis vectors, they will also be at risk if they are responsible for gathering wood in infected areas. Recent studies that have demonstrated that the leishmaniasis sandfly vector inhabits the walls of houses raises issues related to domestic transmission (Kaendi 1994). Women may be more exposed in areas where the disease is highly endemic and vector densities are greater in or near the house (Badaro 1988).

Cysticercosis is an infection produced by larval tapeworms of the genus *Taenia*. It is acquired by eating the raw or undercooked meat of infected pigs and cattle (Sarti 1994). Women's domestic roles may put them at risk of acquiring taeniasis. As they prepare meals, women may eat by nibbling, even when the meat is still raw or undercooked, and can become infected. Moreover, when women prepare and serve food without applying sound sanitary practices, they can become the main sources of cysticercosis to their family if they contaminate the food (Sarti 1994).

The role of women in the promotion and preservation of health in the home also puts them at increased risk of acquiring highly contagious diseases like leprosy and cholera. Women are responsible for caring for ill family members, and the contagious nature of these diseases makes it more likely that they too will contract the diseases (Durana 1994).

> Malaria is a disease of poverty. By and large the rich and powerful live in sanitary surroundings with easy access to medical facilities; whereas, the poor live in crowded urban slums and in remote rural areas that favour transmission. Because ignorance, apathy, and lack of access to medication often prevent them from seeking help early enough, the most serious manifestations of tropical diseases are invariably seen among the underprivileged. Among these, women are particularly vulnerable.
>
> — Rachel Reubin, Centre for Research in Medical Entomology, Madurai, India

DISEASES OF POVERTY

Tropical diseases are "diseases of neglect and exacerbated by poverty" (Amazigo 1994). The impoverished living conditions of many women in the developing world translate into added risk for disease transmission. Many diseases particularly affect those who lack the basic conditions necessary to ensure good health, such as clean water, sanitation, and adequate housing. For example, Bonilla et al. (1991) reported that women living in poor housing and those who fetched water outside the household had more malaria than women who cooked in adequate kitchens or had water in their houses.

Lack of ventilation, poor housing, and overcrowding are risk factors associated with leprosy, a highly infectious disease transmitted through droplets of bodily secretions (from saliva to pus from ulcers) (Duncan 1992). Most cases of leprosy among women in Venezuela were associated with deficient standards of living with regard to economic status (79%), literacy and education (78%), nutrition (75%), hygiene (66%), and living quarters (73%) (Ulrich et al. 1992). Another study found that the prevalence for leprosy in Venezuela was more than six times higher in areas of low economic development than in the areas with the highest levels of development (see Ulrich et al. 1992, p. 12).

The absence of basic systems for sewage disposal and water management at the community level are primary factors that lead to the transmission of cholera. Cholera is an acute, infectious disease of the intestinal tract that is caused when the bacillus *Vibrio cholerae* is swallowed. Humans are believed to be the only reservoir of cholera infection (Stephenson 1987). The parasite is excreted from the body in feces and vomit, and it can be transmitted when patients or infected materials are handled. Flies can also

> As a result of poverty, a high proportion of the Nigerian
> population lives under conditions in which parasitic infections
> thrive. Rural females are disproportionately more disadvantaged.
>
> — Uche Amazigo, Department of Zoology, University of Nigeria,
> Nsukka, Nigeria

carry the parasite to food or water. In Colombia, women living in poor housing constructed over contaminated water and those responsible for fetching water outside the household faced a higher risk of acquiring cholera (Durana 1994).

Chagas' disease is widespread in poor, rural areas throughout Latin America, and women appear to be most adversely affected (Sotomayer et al. 1994). It is caused by infection by the protozoan flagellate parasite *Trypanosoma cruzi* and is most commonly transmitted by bloodsucking triatomine bugs. Traditionally a rural problem, Chagas' disease is increasingly becoming an urban issue as a result of migration. The vector can live and breed in cracks and holes of walls and roofs of poor housing, such as those constructed of mud and thatch. Crowded peri-urban conditions hasten the spread of Chagas' disease, and women living in poverty are most at risk (Sotomayer et al. 1994).

Communities affected by leishmaniasis are often among the most impoverished sectors of a nation (Wijeyaratne et al. 1994). Poor housing and poor hygienic practices increase the risk of transmission of leishmaniasis in peri-domestic areas. The vectors of visceral leishmaniasis are attracted to livestock and dogs kept in the home and to houses made of materials such as grass that are easily invaded by sandflies (WHO 1990). A high number of people sleeping in the same room can also attract sandflies.

> More than half the pregnant women who tested positive for
> Chagas' disease resided beyond the fourth ring, which is an
> economically poor area, [with significant population growth over
> the last decade] that has less access to basic services. There
> was a higher percentage of female heads of households among
> those who tested positive to Chagas' disease.
>
> — Octovio Sotomayer, Dr Percy Boland Maternity Institute, Santa Cruz, Bolivia

The social ostracism women suffer as a result of these diseases is different from that of men. In the case of onchocerciasis and other mutilating diseases, men expect and receive care; whereas women are often shunned by their families, or even banished from their communities and left to die.

— A. El Bindari Hammad, World Health Organization,
Geneva, Switzerland

THE STIGMA OF TROPICAL DISEASE

There is considerable social stigma associated with many tropical diseases for both women and men. Herrin (1988) used a questionnaire to explore the social consequences of schistosomiasis infection in the Philippines. He discovered that people "looked down upon" those who were infected and reported that "it was thought that an individual infected by [schistosomiasis] would damage the social standing of his/her family." Individuals testing positive to Chagas' disease have been denied employment in many Latin American cities and, in Brazil, women infected with Chagas' have lost their jobs when their illness was discovered (Zajac 1992, p. 143).

Leprosy bears a deep historical stigma and is associated with ostracism and sense of fear and revulsion more than any other tropical disease (Ulrich et al. 1992). A study exploring perceptions of those with leprosy found that people were unwilling to employ, work with, provide housing to, or shake hands with leprosy patients (Tekle-Haimanot et al. 1992).

Although stigma can have dramatic personal consequences for both men and women, women can be far more vulnerable because social stigma may compound other problems of powerlessness and subordination that women face simply because they are female (Manderson et al. 1993). A study that explored the implications of disease-related disability on women and men found that a significantly higher percentage of women, compared with men, were divorced with the onset of disability (Hellandendu 1992). Disability affected the woman's chances of staying married depending on the extent to which disability interfered with execution of her household and farming activities (Hellandendu 1992). Because cholera is associated with unsanitary living conditions, men and women afflicted with cholera may be labeled as dirty and poor. Women, who are usually responsible for maintaining healthy living conditions within the home, may feel the shame of such labeling more acutely than men (Durana 1994).

A number of tropical diseases, such as leprosy, guinea worm, leishman-iasis, onchocerciasis, cysticercosis, and urinary schistosomiasis, may cause visible physical disfigurement and disability. Onchocerciasis, for example, can result in a disfiguring skin condition that causes depigmentation and a premature aged appearance (Vlassoff 1994), and leprosy can produce severe mutilation of the face and extremities. Because physical attractiveness is highly valued for women in all societies, and because "[women's] life chances [are] more closely associated with their physical appearance than those of men" (Vlassoff 1994, p. 1251), disfiguring diseases can have a particularly profound impact on women and can generate serious psychological and emotional stress on those afflicted. In a study of leprosy patients in India, 51% of women were forced to leave home because of the disease, compared with 32% of men.[19]

Women with leprosy have been abandoned by their husbands, had their children taken away from them, and even been sent to live in a cave (Mull et al. 1989). Women do not even have to have leprosy themselves to be harmed — they just have to be in contact with infected individuals. Women with male relatives known to have leprosy can have problems marrying (Mull et al. 1989). Almost 70% of nurses in a leprosy-endemic country said that unmarried nurses working in leprosy hospitals would have difficulty getting married (Awofeso 1992).

In some Nigerian communities, leprosy was found to have a devastating impact on the schooling and marriage prospects of girls.[20] Because of complaints from parents of healthy children, teachers expelled infected children. Children who were forced to leave school usually took up menial jobs or quickly married before the onset of physical deformities. Once their condition became visible, adolescent girls with leprosy experienced a high rate of divorce.

Until recently, skin disease associated with onchocerciasis has been given little consideration by disease-control programs — nearly all attention has been on blindness, which is the most debilitating aspect of the disease. However, a study conducted in rural Nigeria found that unsightly lesions from acute and chronic papular dermatitis, and thickened, irritated skin, limited the chances that young adolescent girls would find marriage partners (Amazigo 1994). Girls with this disease also tried to conceal their condition, and often shied away from school and social activities. Stigma not only affected marriage prospects, it also limited the ability to make friends and

---

[19] See Vlassoff, C.; Khot, S.; Rao, S., "Double jeopardy: women and leprosy in India." Unpublished (cited in UN 1995, p. 73).

[20] Unpublished research of M.A. Asuquo, National Institute for Medical Research, PMB 2013, Yaba, Lagos, Nigeria.

Miss A is a 23-year-old unmarried woman who has been treated for onchocerciasis by medical and traditional doctors for 13 of her 23 years. She is physically good looking except for the gross elephantiasis legs. Miss A has never been asked for marriage, and this is attributable to her disfigurement. Miss A now has a 3-month-old baby girl. According to her story, because of the social stigma attached to elephantiasis, and the fear of not being able to have children after a certain age, she fell prey to an old married man and became pregnant from the relationship.

— Uche Amazigo, Department of Zoology, University of Nigeria, Nsukka, Nigeria

"essentially disqualified [those with the disease] from full social acceptance" (Amazigo 1994, p. 88). Males, on the other hand, did not face the same degree of ostracism.

Because some tropical diseases have symptoms that show up in the genital area, they may be incorrectly perceived as STDs. Infected women may be labeled as "immoral," and their disease may be viewed as a "punishment" for sexually promiscuous or deviant behaviour. The sexual freedom accorded to men in most societies, and differential attitudes toward the presence of STDs in men and women, mean that men are generally not treated in such a harsh fashion — indeed, tropical disease symptoms in the genital area can be considered a sign of **virility** for men (Vlassoff and Bonilla 1994). In many African societies, for example, urinary schistosomiasis in men ("red water") is a sign of coming of age and virility.

In Amagunze, Nigeria, schistosomiasis infection in women most frequently affects the urinary system and is regarded by the community as an STD that is associated with immoral sexual behaviour (Amazigo 1994). Hematuria adversely affected the marriage prospects of adolescent girls, led to accusations by husbands of sexual misconduct, caused divorce and abandonment in some cases, and affected women's work capacity and family responsibilities (Amazigo 1994). A woman with urinary schistosomiasis from Anambra State, Nigeria, described her situation (from the 1985 *Nigerian Fertility Survey*, as cited in Amazigo 1994).

> During your adolescent age when other girls are hurrying out of primary school for suitors, you (the infected girl with haematuria) are busy convincing our parents and eligible male friends ... that the blood in your urine is not gonorrhoea contracted from a promiscuous lifestyle. When you finally get married, you complain of (postcoital) bleeding and

irritation in your vagina. Therefore you are unable to satisfy the sexual desires of your husband. Imagine your fate. Even when you are innocent, with these symptoms, who will believe you?

Finally, women are often accused of being the transmitters of disease, and they may be held responsible when other family members fall ill. For example, some people maintain that leprosy is caused by having intercourse with a "bad" or menstruating woman (Mull et al. 1989). Sotomayer et al. (1994) interviewed pregnant women who had tested positive for Chagas' disease in Bolivia. When informed that they had tested positive to Chagas' disease, the women expressed normal fears about dying and the possible detrimental effects to their unborn children; they also expressed a direct concern about the potential reactions of their partners to the news (Sotomayer et al. 1994). Without adequate information, husbands often blame their wives for both the incidence and transmission of Chagas' disease, and warn their children to "be careful of your mother because she may infect you" (Sotomayer et al. 1994, p. 122). This type of reaction caused added stress for the women, who already had to deal with the fact that they were infected.

Health services must be made more aware of the stigmas associated with many tropical diseases, especially for women. More research in this area is needed, particularly about the social and psychological effects (anxiety and depression) of disfigurement for women.

ACCESS TO CARE

The wide range of factors that influence whether or not a woman obtains quality care from available health facilities is discussed in Chapter 8. However, brief mention is made here of some factors because they affect women's access to diagnosis and treatment for tropical diseases.

The overemphasis placed on women's reproductive health in developing countries has had notable negative ramifications for women's care. Because women tend to associate modern health services with family planning or care for their children, they often think that treatment is unavailable for their nonreproductive health needs, and they are therefore hesitant to articulate concerns related to tropical diseases (Vlassoff and Bonilla 1994). A study of women suffering from malaria in Saradidi, Kenya, found that 90% of the women recognized that they were suffering from malaria but 53% did not take prophylaxis because they did not know it was available (Kaseje et al. 1987). Women may not report unusual signs and symptoms because they are "not aware that they (nurses) can treat filariasis. They do not remove nodules and doctors hardly come to our centre" (Amazigo 1994, p. 86). Unfortunately, women's beliefs about available services are usually right. The disproportionate focus on reproduction has resulted in a dearth of personnel and facilities for the detection, documentation, and treatment of tropical diseases among women who attend health-care clinics.

The incredible stigma associated with many tropical diseases also means that women sometimes go to great ends to hide their disease. Women are loathe to expose some of the dreaded effects of lymphatic filariasis and leishmaniasis, which include unsightly deformities in which the legs assume elephantine shape and size. If women perceive themselves to be disfigured or unattractive, they may not feel psychologically prepared to seek treatment. Because they fear rejection and abandonment by friends and family, women often hide their affliction and prefer to remain isolated in their homes, particularly after disease symptoms become visible (Amazigo 1994).

The lack of female health workers can prevent women from presenting for care for all their health needs, and this is particularly the case for physically deforming diseases. The reluctance of women to be seen by male physicians means that early detection of disease is impaired.

The detrimental effects of lymphatic filariasis to the sexual health of Nigerian women would be difficult to document because of the unwillingness of adolescent females and women to undress for the predominantly male health workers or field researchers in Nigeria.

— Uche Amazigo, Department of Zoology, University of Nigeria, Nsukka, Nigeria

---

Although the costs associated with treatment and control of tropical diseases, including insecticide spraying, drug treatment, and hospitalization, can be prohibitive for both men and women, women can be disproportionately hindered by such costs because of the limitations on their earnings and their complete exclusion from the cash economy in some locations (Paolisso and Leslie 1995). With limited financial resources, even relatively low-cost preventive measures such as insecticide-impregnated bednets can be beyond the means of poor households — an inability to afford to buy sufficient nets for all family members, coupled with gender discrimination, can mean that men and boys will be given bednets before women and girls (Alilio 1994).

The various factors impeding women's access to diagnosis and care can make it difficult to confirm definitive sex distributions for tropical diseases. As an illustration, men appear to be more at risk for leprosy than women, and the male to female reported prevalence ratio is about 2 to 1 (Ulrich et al. 1992). Researchers are increasingly suggesting, however, that the accuracy of official statistics could be affected by women's underreporting for care. Limited access to health services, the overburden of household and

> The drug [to treat schistosomiasis] was available in the village
> health centre, at a price of [US] $3 per tablet — equivalent to $12
> per adult dose — which almost none of the villagers could afford.
> This meant that almost no one got treated for their infection.
>
> — Stella Anyangwe, Faculty of Medicine and Biomedical Sciences,
> University of Yaoundé I, Yaoundé, Cameroon

childcare responsibilities, and the stigma associated with leprosy, may make it less likely for women to show up at clinics to be diagnosed and result in gross underestimates of disease prevalence. Even strategies created deliberately to overcome these barriers may be unsuccessful in obtaining accurate numbers. For example, if researchers go from home to home to detect active cases, women in seclusion may be unable to open their doors to males. This could result in the systematic skipping of women (Manderson 1994).

In one rural area of Thailand, there had been a long-held belief that men were more exposed to malaria that women because they showed up at malaria clinics more frequently (only 16% of people attending clinics were women). Survey data, however, revealed no significant sex differences in infection. Furthermore, the introduction of a mobile malaria unit increased women's participation to 33% (Ettling 1989).

WOMEN'S ROLE AS FAMILY HEALTH-CARE PROVIDERS

Illness and disease have special implications for women because, in both developing and industrialized countries, women have a central role as health providers within the family (Jones and Catalan 1989; Strebel 1994). According to gender stereotypes and the sexual division of labour, it is a woman's "natural responsibility" to nurture and take care of household members (Salinas 1988; Lange et al. 1994; Strebel 1994). Women's traditional responsibilities in the promotion and maintenance of the total health and

> According to classical gender stereotypes,
> health care is a woman's role.
>
> — Ilta Lange, School of Nursing, Universidad Católica de Chile, Santiago, Chile

well-being of family members include producing and preparing nutritious foods; providing quality water and essential energy needs; caring for family members, especially children, the disabled, and the elderly; imparting information to others about the prevention and treatment of illnesses and the maintenance of good health; traveling long distances to take children to clinics; treating common diseases and injuries; ensuring the cleanliness of children; undertaking the everyday work of feeding and nursing household members; ensuring sanitation; and trying to keep poor quality housing clean (Momsen 1991; McCauley et al. 1992; Kwawu 1994; Manderson 1994). Women's role as health providers is strongly valued by women themselves (Vlassoff 1994), and even when women have paid work outside the home, they invariably continue to perform these responsibilities.

Women are the actual managers of families and household resources [and] are the nurturers of children and caretakers of spouses.

— Jane Kwawu, Centre for African Family Studies, Nairobi, Kenya

---

Diagnosing illness and caring for the sick

Women are usually the first point of contact when family members are ill (Rathgeber and Vlassoff 1993). Children, if they turn to anyone at all, usually tell their mothers first about their health problems. Mothers also usually diagnose family illnesses, and may "discover ... an infection if they noticed blood on the children's clothing or bed" (Anyangwe et al. 1994, p. 81).

Women do the bulk of the caring for the sick, whereas men rarely take on this responsibility (Tsikata 1994). When a family member is ill, it is a woman who decides whether self-treatment is appropriate, whether and when medical attention is necessary, and what kind of health services are required (Rathgeber and Vlassoff 1993). They may provide a range of products and remedies for treatment of family members, including tonics, herbal extracts, poultices, ointments and oils, and a variety of other medicines

---

A cholera epidemic increases the responsibilities, worries, and work of women.

— Claudia Durana, Faculty of Economics, Universidad do los Andes, Bogotá, Colombia

---

(McCauley et al. 1992; Kettel 1996). Women prepare efficacious herbal remedies for skin diseases, intestinal helminths, constipation, diarrhea, and other complaints (MacCormack 1992). It is women who usually accompany sick family members to a health centre or hospital and act as mediators between health professionals and family members (Cardaci 1992; Tsikata 1994).

[In Simbok], malaria was most often diagnosed by mothers, who, initially, tried traditional remedies such as herbal infusions or a vapour bath over a boiling pot. They then usually proceeded to administer often inadequate doses of various antimalaria medication, especially chloroquine and aspirin, which they purchased without prescriptions.

— Stella Anyangwe, Faculty of Medicine and Biomedical Sciences, University of Yaoundé I, Yaoundé, Cameroon

---

Implications of a woman's illness

There have been few studies measuring the impact of a woman's illness on other family members. It is important that women are healthy both for their own sake and for their key role in maintaining healthy families (Kaendi 1994). The state of women's health and well-being contributes directly to the health and well-being of their families, especially children and the elderly, and therefore contributes to the community as a whole. A woman's incapacitation can affect general family health because she will no longer be able to fill her essential roles (Amazigo 1994; Anyangwe et al. 1994). Incapacitation as a result of malaria, for example, prevents women from taking advantage of antenatal services and from taking infants to clinics for immunization (Brieger et al. 1989).

Chronic and repeated malaria infections, or serious schistosomiasis infection, can lead to decreased capacity for women to carry out their household and farming activities. A household will probably experience a loss of income during a woman's illness if she is involved in the paid work force

---

Losses caused by Chagas' disease of women in endemic areas may substantially alter the economic status of entire communities.

— Octavio Sotomayer, Dr Percy Boland Maternity Institute, Santa Cruz, Bolivia

---

(Durana 1994). However, loss of income caused by illness can be difficult to measure because women who suffer from disease may work longer hours or work even harder just to meet the demands of their job.

If a woman is very ill and experiences great pain or is hospitalized, her domestic and economic work must still be done, which can have negative implications for other family members, particularly in female-headed households. A World Bank study found that school attendance of young people aged 15–20 years was reduced by half if the household had lost an adult female member in the previous year (World Bank 1993). Girls are particularly affected and are more likely than boys to be kept from schooling to assume increased domestic responsibilities in societies where girls' education is given lower priority than boys' (WASH Field Report 1988; World Bank 1993). In the case of serious maternal illness, "the mother's burden becomes the daughter's sacrifice — a sacrifice much less frequently demanded of boys" (UNFPA 1990, p. 15). More research to explore the effects of a woman's illness is needed, particularly its effects on absenteeism, drop-out rates, and learning outcomes of school-age girls (Amazigo 1994; Anyangwe et al. 1994).

> There are no studies that examine the social and economic consequences of blindness [stemming from onchocerciasis] on women's domestic and economic roles, particularly among female-headed households. Blindness of a mother may have a disastrous effect on the family.
>
> — Uche Amazigo, Department of Zoology, University of Nigeria, Nsukka, Nigeria

Disease-control measures

Many diseases are transmitted either within or around the household and can best be controlled by careful management of the local biophysical environment. Control strategies consequently must involve the active participation of all householders. The social role of women as health providers within the family provides them with opportunities to play an important role in controlling the transmission of disease at the household level. Indeed, the ultimate success and effectiveness of interventions may depend on the participation of women.

Women have significant power and authority within the domestic domain. If women's cooperation is not assured in interventions, there may be low rates of participation in disease-control activities. For example, if women

Women had the main responsibility of carrying out cholera-prevention measures in the household: boiling water, cleaning the inside and around the house, and taking care of the children.

— Claudia Durana, Faculty of Economics, Universidad do los Andes, Bogotá, Colombia

are uncomfortable with the intrusion of male vector-control personnel into their household, they may resist the reorganization of the domestic environment to fit control measures.

A good example of the importance of gaining the compliance and cooperation of women to ensure the success of interventions can be seen in the case of bednets. Insecticide-impregnated bednets are increasingly being used as a control strategy for malaria in Asia, Latin America, and Africa. Nets soaked in antimosquito insecticide and used to cover beds can significantly reduce malaria-related deaths (WHO 1993). Women will probably bear the primary responsibility for reimpregnating bed nets every 6 months, and the success of this intervention will depend on their participation (Alilio 1994; Amazigo 1994).

As described by (Reubin 1992, p. 49) in *Women and Tropical Diseases*:

> It is [women] who will bring the family bed nets to the health centres to be dipped in pyrethroid suspension, it is they who will put them on mattresses to dry, and see that the children stay under them at night. It is they who will decide whether the nets are to be washed and at what intervals, and when they need to be retreated with pyrethroid because mosquitoes are beginning to bite again. Similarly, if mosquito repellent creams, soaps, or smokes are used on a large scale in integrated control programmes of the future, it will be the responsibility of the women to see that they are used properly by the family, and that children in particular wash repellent applications off their skins before reapplication

Vlassoff (1994) reported that a pilot study funded by WHO in Ghana sought to determine people's preferences for insecticide-impregnated bednets. They found that women did not want white nets because they quickly became dirty and unsightly. As a result, a decision was made to dye the nets gray. To date, the project has proceeded well.

Sanitary conditions are the key to preventing diseases such as leishmaniasis, cysticercosis, and cholera. Because women usually have major responsibility for household sanitation and environmental practices, their participation in any control and treatment strategy is clearly essential to ensure its sustainability. Women can play an important role in strategies to improve sanitation and hygiene practices, such as ensuring proper garbage disposal and drainage, improving the quality of the water supply, adopting hygienic food-preparation practices, and eliminating actual or potential sandfly breeding and resting sites, such as garbage piles, piles of bricks, and stones (Stephenson 1987; Warren et al. 1993).

Education of family members on health

The full participation of women in the process of health education is important. Women in most cultures play an important role in informing family members about health beliefs, illness behaviour, and the use of health services. They can, therefore, play a crucial role in the prevention and control of disease. For example, women educate their children about personal hygiene habits and health practices — such as brushing teeth, food consumption and nutrition, and the importance of proper sanitation and waste disposal — and ensure that children are immunized and cared for during the crucial years (Kwawu 1994; Lule and Ssembatya 1995). Women who are properly educated about tropical diseases can educate children about the parasite, routes of infection, and development of disease.

Because education efforts focused mainly on women not only improve their health, but also the health of their families, interventions are increasingly targeting mothers to produce changes in health-related practices (Sarti 1994). Women who have been encouraged to change from an old water source to a new one, or who have been persuaded to use a latrine maintained by the household rather than to defecate in the bush can educate other family members about the importance of these practices. To reduce the transmission of schistosomiasis, women can be encouraged to limit their contact with infested waters and to teach their children not to play in infected lakes. As observed by Yudomustopo (1995) in Indonesia:

> Children who lived alongside the river enjoyed playing, bathing, and even toileting in the river. Women as mothers and educators took responsibility for the safety of their children ... and most women forbade their children from these activities.

Mata (1982) found that in a Mayan Indian village maternal attitudes and practices had greater impact on disease transmission in the family than socioeconomic class or level of education. Sarti (1994) from the Dirección Nacional de Epidemiologia, Secretaría de Salud, Mexico, produced changes in hygienic and sanitary practices related to disease through programs of community education focused on mothers. The mothers then went on to teach their children preventive health practices.

Although women's role as providers of family health must be respected and taken into consideration in interventions, researchers have also been quick to point out the drawbacks of exclusively targeting women in disease-control interventions. Rathgeber and Vlassoff (1993), for example, cautioned that a focus on women as health providers may reinforce the notion that women are responsible for failures in disease-control efforts at the community level and lead to criticisms of women if desired activities are not implemented. Women may also need to make significant investments of time and energy to carry out the recommended control measures, and this could lead to the further overburdening of women (Winch et al. 1994). In this regard, there is a need for research to explore strategies that might lead to a more equitable distribution of family roles. Although the importance of gaining women's cooperation in disease-control measures must be remembered, family-health messages should perhaps be targeted at both women and men, rather than be directed solely to women (which perpetuates the idea that family health is primarily or exclusively the responsibility of women). Men must be encouraged to take a more active role in creating and maintaining a healthy home environment rather than to leave the entire responsibility to women.

Health messages directed to women can perpetuate the idea that family health is primarily or exclusively the responsibility of women.

— Ilta Lange, School of Nursing, Universidad Católica de Chile, Santiago, Chile

Knowledge levels

The ability of women to protect themselves from disease and to properly educate family members about prevention and treatment strategies is contingent
on their access to proper information. Much research, however, points to significant gaps in women's understanding of disease. In Baringo, Kenya, significantly fewer women (12%) than men (26%) knew the correct etiology of
visceral leishmaniasis (Kaendi 1994). Women's capacity to protect themselves and their families is hindered by a lack of understanding of causes,
symptoms, transmission routes, and prevention and treatment strategies.

A study of the transmission of malaria among adolescent girls in rural
Ghana found that malaria was often believed to be caused by excessive heat
and that most community members did not connect malaria to mosquitos
(see Agyepong 1992). Although most women understood that malaria was
caused by mosquito bites in a study conducted in Cameroon, some reported
other causes including heavy rains, walking for a long time under the sun,
and catching a cold (Anyangwe et al. 1994). In the same study, most mothers stopped giving malaria treatment to their children when the fever sub-
sided, even if it was after a single dose of medication.

In the Philippines, women sometimes put themselves at risk of malaria
because they were unaware of the risks (Espino 1995). One mother would
constantly go out of the mosquito net at night to prepare milk for her young
infant. One pregnant woman refused treatment because she believed it
would harm the baby. After she had given birth, this woman was diagnosed
with malaria, but she gave the prescribed medication to the infant because
she believed the baby had malaria (Espino 1995).

There were serious misconceptions among women in Cameroon about
how schistosomiasis was acquired. Women thought that the "worms" that
cause schistosomiasis entered the human body through the urethra or anus
during urination or defecation in the lake (Anyangwe et al. 1994). In Peru,
women frequently attributed leishmaniasis to "contact with stale water, contact with the morning dew, and contact with the toroq tree, mosquitos and
butterflies" (Timoteo and Llanos-Cuentas 1994, p. 129).

Many women in endemic areas lack information about Chagas' disease
(Zajac 1992; Sotomayer et al. 1994). In a study conducted in rural Bolivia,
59% of women did not realize that triatomine bugs transmitted Chagas' disease, although they recognized the bugs and had seen them in their homes
(see Zajac 1992).

Superstitious beliefs about other diseases have also been reported.
Some women in Colombia thought cholera was a "disease of fate" (Durana
1994); whereas, leishmaniasis in Kosnipata, Peru, was sometimes attributed
to magic or a retribution from God (Timoteo and Llanos-Cuentas 1994).

One of the primary risk factors of Chagas' infection for women of low socioeconomic status is the lack of information about Chagas' disease and the way it is transmitted. Much of the information about the disease is based on speculation or mythical beliefs [and some] pregnant women believed they are subject to witchcraft, sorcery, or some evil spell, or are infected by another person.

— Octovio Sotomayer, Dr Percy Boland Maternity Institute, Santa Cruz, Bolivia

The decision-making authority of men

Many researchers have also pointed out that interventions that exclusively target women because they are responsible for the care of children may have little impact because men have so much decision-making power within households (Amazigo 1994; Chiarella 1994; Kaendi 1994; Vlassoff 1994; Bello 1995; Udipi and Varghese 1995). In some cultures, women are expected to make decisions about child-health matters without necessarily involving other family members; however, in other societies, "the decision to change behaviour ha[s] to be sanctioned by the husband in the household and the community as a whole" (McCauley et al. 1992). In one study, permission to attend meetings with groups of women was often granted only after the goals of the program had been explained to community members and husbands (McCauley et al. 1992). According to a woman from KwaZulu-Natal, South Africa, "we need our husband's permission for absolutely everything" (Pagé 1995, p. 8).

In the case of activities to prevent malaria, for example, the male of the household may make the crucial and ultimate decision concerning whether or not a mosquito net will be used, and if so, by which family

In Simbok, fathers made the decision about when to go to a health-care facility for treatment. Mothers had to ask fathers for money and permission to take themselves or their children to the health centre if they deemed the infection serious enough to require treatment.

— Stella Anyangwe, Faculty of Medicine and Biomedical Sciences, University of Yaoundé I, Yaoundé, Cameroon

members. Fathers, and sometimes mothers-in-law, may decide whether malaria prophylactics will be used. Mothers-in-law have reportedly prevented their daughters-in-law from taking malaria prophylactics because they believed they were in fact oral contraceptives (WHO 1995). According to Rogler (1989, cited in Yack 1992), interventions based on the assumption that mothers have the freedom to make health-care decisions for their children, presupposes the existence of a situation of choices, with mothers and significant others bidding for their preferences, within the context of equal say in households.

The adequate use of health services is intertwined with gender inequality. Women of low socioeconomic status cannot make a unilateral decision to seek health care. The decision is made either by the spouse or mother-in-law.

— Trinidad S. Osteria, De La Salle University, Manila, Philippines

A study conducted by Halima Abdullah Mwenesi, from the Kenya Medical Research Centre, Nairobi, Kenya, provided a clear example of women's relative lack of decision-making power in some societies. Mwenesi examined the decision-making dynamics with regard to health-seeking behaviour among the Mijikenda and the Luo peoples of the Kilifi District, Coast Province, Kenya. She reported that both Luo and Mijikenda mothers, following the dictates of their patriarchal societies, are not expected to make any decision concerning themselves or their (husband's) children without consulting their husbands or other males in the household (Mwenesi 1994). Women routinely consulted their husband, and, in the absence of the husband, his father and brothers. Only if the father was away and the husband's brothers were younger siblings, would senior females in the household — usually the mother-in-law or a senior sister-in-law — be consulted.

These societies have a well-defined social structure in which everyone "knows their place" (Mwenesi 1994). Husbands are consulted because "it is the way it is" (Mwenesi 1994), and men make all financial decisions. Among the Luo people, if relationships of seniority are ignored, it is believed that the "chira" infliction will befall the household. Qualitative research from male and female informants revealed that women could decide on simple home remedies or purchase over-the-counter drugs (such as acetylsalicylic acid, ASA). However, someone other than the mother had to be involved in important matters such as whether or not to seek treatment at a health facility or from a traditional healer, because it was believed that the husband (or his stand-ins) would be able to make a wiser decision than the mother.

*Almost all mothers, 880 out of 883, sought advice before
taking an ill child to a hospital.*

— Halima Abdullah Mwenesi, Kenya Medical Research Institute, Nairobi, Kenya

Similarly, McCauley et al. (1992) reported that, among the Gogo people of Tanzania, mothers were responsible for the care of their ill children and treated them with herbal teas for minor ailments, but they had to seek the express permission of their husbands before using a health facility or traditional healer. Similar findings from Zaire were reported by Janzen (1978). The implications of these findings are serious — "the time taken to consult various people for a child suffering from a severe disease could mean death or severe impairment" (Mwenesi 1994, p. 124). Likewise, if the woman herself is ill, her health could also be placed in jeopardy by such delays.

Although interventions should recognize the importance of women as health promoters at the family level, they must also be sensitive to the complex set of factors that influence health behaviours. Women's lower status in the family must be considered, as must the fact that ultimate decision-making authority within households may rest with men. There is much work to be done with regard to improving the position of women in developing societies before exclusively women-centred interventions can be viewed as feasible solutions (Kaendi 1994).

*[Women had to consult husbands because] husbands were
suspicious of health-facility visits and believed that women
sometimes used the children's illnesses or "Well Baby Clinic"
visits as an excuse to go to health facilities for family-planning
services. Most male informants did not see the
need for these services.*

— Halima Abdullah Mwenesi, Kenya Medical Research Institute, Nairobi, Kenya

Chapter 7

Barriers to Quality Health Care

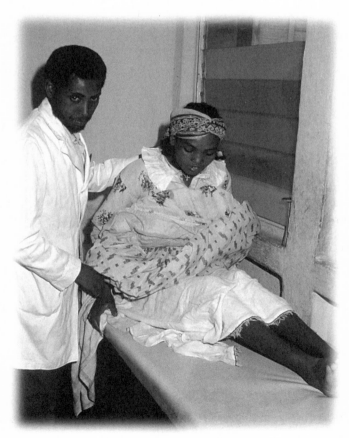

IDRC: D. Marchand

> A gender analysis can provide a perspective on the structure of
> health services, their performance, and delivery. The ability of
> health systems to provide for, and differentiate between, gender
> needs is a test of their relevance and purpose. [These]
> perspectives are required to analyze the changes that
> face — some would say threaten — health institutions
> and practices in developing countries.
>
> — A.D. Tillett, International Development Research Centre, Regional Office for
> Latin America and the Caribbean, Montevideo, Uruguay

There are an extremely wide range of factors that influence whether or not a woman seeks and obtains quality care from modern health-care facilities. The obstacles that women face are much "more than a problem of distance" (Timyan et al. 1993, p. 217) and a lack of financial resources to cover the cost of care and transportation (although these are certainly important factors).

Literature in this area tends to distinguish between "access to care" and "quality of care." Quality-of-care research usually centres on the experiences of those who have managed to gain access to modern health services, but the individuals who choose not to use services, or who are unable to do so, are not addressed. However, female clients may consider access to care to be integrally linked to quality of care (Ndhlovu 1994); conversely, services considered to be of poor quality will not be used. Therefore, barriers that influence whether or not a woman is able to gain access to services will be addressed, as will factors that influence the quality of care provided to women at the point of service delivery.

RECOGNITION OF ILLNESS

Before a woman decides to seek care, she must be able to recognize the signs and symptoms that indicate the need for care (AbouZahr 1994; Manderson 1994). However, a lack of educational opportunities and poor understanding of health-related matters mean that many women are not familiar with different diseases and their presentation. For example, some women assume that "vaginal discharge is a natural part of being a woman" (Pesce 1994, p. 19) or think that back pain is normal because they have suffered from it for as long as they can remember.

*How many girls and women in the world still suffer from poverty
of education, information, and knowledge? This type of poverty
denies women the understanding of how their bodies function, how
they can protect themselves, and how to prevent diseases.*

— A. El Bindari Hammad, World Health Organization, Geneva, Switzerland

As a result of cultural restrictions and taboos, women may be unable
to interpret signs of illness, particularly as they relate to the genitals.
Manneschmidt (see footnote 6), for example, reported that "there is a collective denial of women's sexual issues in Nepalese society," and this has led
to the absence of Nepali terms to describe aspects of the female genitals and
gynecological symptoms. Manderson (1994) described how some women,
who lack knowledge about the workings of their bodies, are unable to differ-
entiate normal menstrual blood from other sources of blood (such as blood
in the urine from schistosomiasis), especially in cases where genital mutilation has occurred. Manderson also explained that some women may not even
notice the occurrence of minor bleeding (for example, if they urinate and
bathe while clothed, as some cultural practices demand).

COMPETING DEMANDS

Even if a woman notices symptoms of illness, she may completely ignore
these signs because of other competing demands. Women may believe that
they cannot afford the "luxury" to take time out to visit a health centre or to
have a period of incapacity because this would represent time and effort lost
to other essential, and possibly more important, activities such as child care,
food production, and paid employment (AbouZahr 1994; Bhattacharyya and
Hati 1995). Temporary female workers in the Chilean fruit-picking industry,
for example, said that their long working days made it impossible for them to
leave their work to attend to their health problems (Berr 1994).

*When women suffer from conditions such as infections of the
reproductive tract or tuberculosis, they often deny their
symptoms until they are too serious or too severe to ignore
because of heavy competing workloads.*

— A. El Bindari Hammad, World Health Organization, Geneva, Switzerland

Because they were responsible for the well-being of their families, women living in extreme poverty in Montevideo, Uruguay, said "[they were] not able to leave their children alone" and "what should I go and seek the doctor for, I waste time" (Bonino 1994, p. 201). Women from Chad reported that they were unable to take a sick child for care because "[w]e've got other children at home waiting for us. They have to go to school and we have to go the market" (Wyss and Nandjingar 1995, p. 148).

> Generally, mothers say that they are busy, that they are not able to come [to the health centre], that they have to travel or that they are traders. They also say that their business nourishes the whole family and they cannot neglect all the children just for one.
> — Kasper Wyss and Monique Nandjingar, Swiss Tropical Institute, Basel, Switzerland

The hours when health clinics are open may not be sensitive to the gender division of labour and the timing of women's work. As a result of the daytime responsibilities of women — such as fetching water, feeding chickens, collecting the firewood, and going to the factory — it might be easier for women to visit clinics in the evening instead of in the daytime when modern health services are usually open. Women's work patterns should therefore be considered when setting clinic hours. To increase the chances of working women receiving care, health services might also be established where women work, such as at factories (MacCormack 1992).

Other family or community members rarely assume women's essential tasks when they are ill. Women therefore continue to perform necessary activities that are difficult to defer (Watts et al. 1989; Bonilla et al. 1991). Because women do not take off enough time to care for their health, it usually takes them longer to fully recover from illness or disease. The amount of time that a woman stays in hospital (if she has to go) can be significantly shorter than the amount of time taken by a man (Bhattacharyya and Hati 1995), and a woman invariably returns to her work, both inside and outside the home, before she is fully recovered.

> Women are unwilling to go to service points for their own health because their absence will disrupt household and economic activities.
> — Trinidad S. Osteria, De La Salle University, Manila, Philippines

*A woman's everyday routine is full of small waivers of herself
that are acts of giving herself up to others.*

— Constanza Collazos V., Centro de Investigaciones
Multidisciplinarias en Desarrollo, Cali, Colombia

WOMEN'S HEALTH IS NOT A PRIORITY

Women in developing countries tend to place the health and well-being of their families, especially children, as a priority over their own health and, consequently, do not seek medical care for themselves. Women "give everything to [their] children" because "the children always come first" and "the only thing [they] have in life is [their] children" (Bonino 1994, p. 201). Women will ignore their own symptoms of disease and illness, but always go "to the pregnancy check-ups as a duty, because ... it is a duty to do it for the welfare of the child" (Bonino 1994, p. 202). Furthermore, male children tend to be given superior access to care compared with female children (Chatterjee 1990). In a study conducted in Bangladesh, male children less than 5 years old were brought to a treatment facility for diarrhea illness more frequently than females — the male use rate was 66% higher than the female use rate (Chen et al. 1981).

The general low status of women, and their internalization of this status, results in the marginalization of women's physical, psychological, and emotional needs (Kwawu 1994; Manderson 1994; Bhattacharyya and Hati 1995). Women are less likely than men to consult modern health services, wait longer than men to seek treatment when ill, are reluctant to spend limited resources on their own needs, and often cope with illness by self-treatment, by consulting traditional healers, or by simply living with the condition and its resulting discomfort (Mechanic 1976; Lorber 1984; Rathgeber and Vlassoff 1993; Kwawu 1994; Iqbal 1995).

*Because of their heavy household duties, women cannot afford
to be sick themselves. It would be useful to discover how many
ailments exist among women but never receive attention from
the medical profession.*

— Dzodzi Tsikata, Institute of Statistical, Social and Economic Research,
University of Ghana, Legon, Ghana

A leader of a very poor community outside of Montevideo, Uruguay, reported that, "[a] women here does not take care of herself at all. The husband or the children always come first, for the children she does have time" (Bonino 1994, p. 201). One woman from the same study reported that "I think that we give more importance to our children than to ourselves" (p. 202).

Women associate the use of a dispensary, clinic, or hospital services with the health of their children (Kwawu 1994) and generally attend health centres primarily to obtain care for their children, although they may also be suffering from a health problem. Iqbal (1995) reported that it was "observed many times that a woman who comes ... worrying about her child was herself suffering from some disease, mostly anemia and malnutrition." In an onchocerciasis hyperendemic community in Enegu State, Nigeria, women who came to the only health centre in the community were asked on three occasions their reasons for attending the clinic (Amazigo 1994). Of the 53 women (16–39 years old) asked about their reasons for attending a primary health-care program, 47 came because their children were sick, 5 women came because they were pregnant, and 1 had fever and diarrhea. Nevertheless, 20 (38%) of these women had at least one clinical manifestation of onchocerciasis.

When asked why she was not presenting her own health needs along with those of her children, a respondent observed: "The services here [at the health centre] are for our children and diseases that affect them [poliomyelitis, tetanus, tuberculosis, and measles]. I am not aware that they [the nurses] can treat filariasis. They do not remove nodules and doctors hardly come to our centre.

— Uche Amazigo, University of Nigeria, Nsukka, Nigeria

Women need to be broadly educated about the importance of regular health care for themselves, as well as for their children. The role of self-esteem, an important factor that affects whether or not women seek care for their own health, should be considered when educational health programs are implemented (Bonino 1994). Because women tend to place great importance on their children, it may be useful to present messages that instill the notion that it is important that a woman be healthy to maintain her child's health (Iqbal 1995).

To take care of her own health, [a woman must] recognize herself as an individual, find herself worthy, strengthen her self-esteem, and [have] the power to decide about her own health.

— Constanza Collazos V., Centro de Investigaciones
Multidisciplinarias en Desarrollo, Cali, Colombia

LACK OF SUPPORT

Social support from others, such as relatives, friends, and neighbours can play an important role in fostering the physical and psychological health of women (Bonino 1994), and can greatly influence the health-seeking behaviour of women. Many women, particularly poor women, and those solely responsible for the care of their households, "lack the support of the family, someone to tell her to go to the doctor, to take care of herself, no one worries about her" (Bonino 1994, p. 204). Less importance may be placed on the health of female members of the household, compared with male members, and, consequently, a woman's illness may receive little attention from others (Bhattacharyya and Hati 1995). Although men are strongly pressured by other family members, particularly from mothers and wives, to seek treatment, women are unlikely to receive such encouragement (Niraula 1994) — "a woman's role is to nurse, not to be nursed."

A study conducted in an Egyptian hamlet found that a sick person's access to care was determined by the persons's status within the family. Young women, considered to be of low-status, were likely to be treated by home remedies or traditional healers. "The women seem[ed] to need to convince the men that they [were] dangerously ill before they [were] taken to the doctor" (Lane and Meleis 1991, p. 1206). However, individuals with higher status, such as men of all ages and adult mothers of sons, were likely to be taken directly to a private medical practitioner.

[A woman] needs to be told to go for her own good and needs someone to support her at all times. What happen[ed] is that I went to the hospital by myself, I had no one to take me, so I stopped going.

— Quoted by Maria Bonino, Universidad de la República,
Montevideo, Uruguay

The true extent of some women's health problems may be completely underestimated by society. Paolisso and Leslie (1995) pointed out that, because some very serious illnesses and conditions may not be properly acknowledged by society (for example, cancer, AIDS, physical disabilities, chronic fatigue, and depression), women with such problems may not be assigned "a legitimate sick status." If a woman's illness is not identified as being authentic, it is doubtful that she will receive support from family members and the wider community to seek care.

SHAME AND EMBARRASSMENT

Shame and embarrassment can lead to a reluctance on the part of women to share disease conditions with family members and health providers (Bhattacharyya and Hati 1995; Lule and Ssembatya 1995), and this may prevent them from reporting to health services for the diagnosis and treatment of illnesses. A reluctance to tell others is particularly acute in the case of illnesses with genital or urinary involvement (Amazigo 1994; Manderson 1994). There is considerable stigma associated with STDs because these diseases are associated with sexual deviance. It is not surprising that women are very concerned about the consequences of detection and the possibility of being ostracized by their family and community (Guimarães 1994; Lule and Ssembatya 1995). Vlassoff (1994) also pointed out that women who have been victims of violence and abuse may be very unwilling to seek medical care because they are reluctant to draw attention to their situation.

Health services must be sensitive to the shame and embarrassment many women associate with illnesses. For example, if the stigma associated with STDs were recognized, health services could improve the prospects that women would seek care by offering multiple services that ensure private consultations so that it is not obvious why a person is visiting the centre (World Bank 1993).

FEAR OF ILLNESS

In a qualitative study of women in a very poor area outside of Montevideo, Uruguay, Bonino (1994) documented many of the fears that women may have that prevent them from visiting health centres for care. Some women expressed concern that diseases would be discovered during check-ups and they said "they would rather not know [about them]." One woman was concerned that she might have "cancer of the uterus" and she would "rather not know" because her "mother-in-law died of cancer of the uterus" and her "sister-in-law left behind five children, she died of cancer of the uterus." The inclusion of blood tests in regular check-ups may lead to other concerns. According to one woman, "if they are going to do the HIV, I'm not going — what if I've got AIDS?" (Bonino 1994, p. 202)

APATHY AND DEPRESSION

Women who suffer from psychological conditions, such as depression, may have a complete sense of apathy toward their own health care (Bonino 1994). Although psychological conditions often have a biological component, the particularly harsh living conditions of many women, including poverty, high stress, isolation, and an absence of social support, may work together to produce a state of depression or apathy (Bernardi and Mouriño 1991). The inability of some women to express their problems may adversely affect their psychological health. For other women, childhood experiences of violence, including rape or incest, may be factors related to their apathy or depression (Ferrando 1992). An American study (Joyce 1988) reviewed the histories of 70 women who had not had prenatal care. The study concluded that the psychosocial barriers of depression, negation, and fears were more powerful deterrents to the use of prenatal care than external barriers such as the lack of medical insurance or transport.

ACCESS TO HEALTH FACILITIES

People should be able to receive reliable care close to where they live. However, health facilities are often poorly distributed, and health personnel and financial resources tend to be concentrated in urban hospitals (World Bank 1993; Atai-Okei 1994). Rural areas, where the vast majority of women in the developing world live, are less likely to have adequate health services.

In Kabugao, Philippines, a community in Kalinga-Apayao Province that suffers one of the highest prevalence rates of malaria in the country, the district hospital and rural clinic are reached by boat or half a day's hike through the mountain. The better-equipped provincial hospital is almost a one day journey by jeep. During the peak of the rainy season, the river becomes impossible to cross.

— Esperanzo Espino, Department of Parasitology and Medical Entomology, Research Institute for Tropical Medicine, Manila, Philippines

Difficulties in reaching health facilities, as a result of distances, lack of transportation, or poor roads, are well-documented impediments to care (World Bank 1993; Atai-Okei 1994; Kaendi 1994; Iqbal 1995; Ren et al. 1995). In a study on malaria and visceral leishmaniasis that took place in Baringo, Kenya, during 1992–93, Kaendi (1994) found that distance was the major determining factor in the use of health care. Gender differences were reported, and 62% of the women (compared with 48% of the men) indicated that distance influenced their health-seeking behaviour. Malaria can be a serious problem where there is no health-care facility — "many ... have died of illness before getting to hospital" (Anyangwe et al. 1994, p. 78).

In a study of 390 women who attended an antenatal clinic at Nankumba Health Centre, Mangochi District, Malawi (Lule and Ssembatya 1995), distance to the health centre was the primary reason reported by women to explain why less than one-quarter of the women delivered at a health centre, although almost 90% wanted to. The researchers reported that the number of mothers who delivered at the health centre was indirectly related to the distance in kilometres from the health centre. Of mothers who lived within 1 kilometre of the health centre, 90% delivered their babies there; whereas, only 10% of those who lived more than 20 kilometres away used the health centre. Similarly, distance from the health centre also heavily influenced the number of mothers who presented for care in their second and third stages of pregnancy.

Rodney (1995) reported that Grenadian women identified the lack of transportation as one of the primary barriers to services, particularly in the rural areas. They claimed there was a shortage of state-owned transportation in certain areas and that the privately owned minibuses targeted the high-density urban areas.

There are a number of major problems with the state and private community health centres [in Cambodia]. Health centres are sparsely distributed and good facilities are usually too far away. There is always a lack of transportation. Security is poor and there are safety risks associated with travelling to health centres at night. Because of the lack of infrastructure, sick people often do not arrive at health centres in time for proper treatment.

— Neang Ren, Cambodian Midwives Association, Phnom Penh, Cambodia

In rural areas, the common mode of transportation for women is walking (or occasionally a bicycle). If an ill woman wants to visit a health centre, she may have to walk very long distances. If her child is ill, she may have to walk several kilometres with the sick child strapped on her back (Kaendi

Clients who are farther away are less likely to have a good understanding or an exposure to the services provided by the facility. Greater familiarity can bring with it higher levels of acceptability.

— W. Bailey, Department of Geography, University of West Indies, Jamaica

1994). These long distances often mean that women only visit clinics when their health, or the health of their child, has reached a critical stage (Lule and Ssembatya 1995).

Bailey et al. (1995, p. 333) pointed out that the negative correlation between distance and the use of medical facilities is not always strictly related to the "friction of distance" — it can also be linked women's degree of familiarity with services.

Health facilities must be made more accessible if their use in the prevention and control of disease and illness is to be encouraged (Kaendi 1994). Mobile clinics or the provision of transportation might greatly improve accessibility for women (UN 1995).

RESTRICTIONS ON MOBILITY

Cultural norms that restrict the movements of women in some societies can prevent women from consulting health services (Leslie 1992; Rathgeber and Vlassoff 1993; Manderson 1994; Udipi and Varghese 1995). In rural areas of Pakistan, for example, females are not allowed to travel long distances alone. A male member of the family, even the youngest brother or son, is required to accompany a woman (Iqbal 1995). In Nigeria, "the religious practice of *purdah* severely restricts women's interactions with men and strangers. This limits the distance women can travel alone to seek health care" (Paolisso and Leslie 1995, p. 61). To get around this barrier to care, MacCormack (1992, p. 834) suggested that "elderly widows of secure honour and status might be trained as health workers to visit women in domestic seclusion."

When women are prevented from enjoying their legal, social, and cultural rights, they are disadvantaged with regard to access to health care.

— Trinidad S. Osteria, De La Salle University, Manila, Philippines

> *A woman-centred strategy would require additional measures such as encouraging female community nurses to visit homes, especially those in communities where women are in seclusion, for case detection and management as part of the program to control malaria.*
>
> — Uche Amazigo, Department of Zoology, University of Nigeria, Nsukka, Nigeria

ACCESS TO FINANCIAL RESOURCES

Lack of access to resources to cover transport, service, and treatment costs is another barrier to care (Chiarella 1994; Bhattacharyya and Hati 1995). Women generally lack control of financial resources (often scarce) and therefore cannot, or will not, divert them for their own health. Paolisso and Leslie (1995, p. 61) state

> Given the limitations on women's earnings in both formal and informal employment, and their complete exclusion from the cash economy in some cases, the extent to which poor women, particularly those who head households, can afford expenditures [associated with health care] is questionable.

Because they are financially dependent on husbands or relatives (Mwenesi 1994), women rely on male household members to pay the costs associated with health services. Men usually have the ultimate financial decision-making power about whether or not a family member can go to a health centre (Anyangwe et al. 1994; Kaendi 1994; Tsikata 1994; Vlassoff 1994).

> *Among the Mijikenda people, women are perceived to be the property of men because men pay a dowry to marry. Women are not expected to make any decisions without consulting their husbands. Illnesses, whatever their nature, are [perceived to be] a matter of life and death, and such matters cannot be left in the hands of women. Someone other than the mother must be involved in the health-seeking process. Mothers [also] require financial assistance to pay for either the treatment or the transport, and very few have their own money.*
>
> — Halima Abdullah Mwenesi, Kenya Medical Research Institute, Nairobi, Kenya

Qualitative research results clearly describe the financial difficulties faced by women. A woman from Chad said: "Every time you have to pay 100 francs for this, 100 francs for that. If you multiply these 100 francs by the number of times you go to the hospital, you are not able to find the necessary money" (Wyss and Nandjingar 1995, p. 144). A similar sentiment was expressed by a woman from Kenya: "I have heard that here ... services are not free ... so if you do not have, for example, 20 shillings, [you] cannot get the services" (Ndhlovu 1994, p. 12). Another woman from Kenya complained about the cost of transportation: "She was going to take me to Kenyatta National Hospital ... but I need[ed] to find money for bus fare and I did not have this. So we did not go" (Ndhlovu 1994, p. 11).

Focus-group discussions conducted with adolescent girls in the slum revealed that they did not trust government hospital services. The general opinion was that health [care] is not affordable to the poor.

— S.A. Udipi and M.A. Varghese, SNDT Women's University, Bombay, India

---

As transitional economies, such as those in Cambodia, China, Laos, Mongolia, and Viet Nam, move from centrally planned economies under socialist governments to market economies, user fees are increasingly being introduced and more and more men and women are having to pay for essential health services. Zhang (1994), from the Department of Public Health, Kunming Medical College, China, reported that economic reforms and the introduction of user fees have made services less accessible for some women. A number of disadvantaged women from very poor households who used to enjoy free services may now be unable to see a rural doctor when necessary. Because employment opportunities are not equally available to women and men, women are more disadvantaged by having to pay for health services.

Their treatment-seeking behaviour had more to do with their lack of financial resources than with their lack of will or knowledge to seek treatment.

— Stella Anyangwe, Faculty of Medicine and Biomedical Sciences, University of Yaoundé I, Yaoundé, Cameroon

---

SEX AND MATURITY OF THE
HEALTH WORKER

In many poor countries, the primary health-care worker is male. The lack of female health-care providers is another deterrent that prevents women from reporting to health services, particularly for illnesses involving the genitals and those causing physical deformities. When female clients do see male providers, shyness and reservation, especially concerning sexual health matters, can make it nearly impossible to establish a good client–provider relationship (Iqbal 1995; Manneschmidt, see footnote 6).

Cultural dictates may simply not allow women to be seen by male providers. In some Middle Eastern countries, for example, most physicians are men; however, there is a strong cultural belief that women should not be seen after puberty by men who are not part of their family (World Bank 1993). In Bangladesh, ideologies of purity and shame are so important to the status of women that Muslim female patients cannot speak directly to their doctors; instead, husbands or fathers explain the women's health concerns to the doctor on their behalf (Rozario 1995). A female care provider is preferred to a male for obstetrical and gynaecological care in Pakistan, even if the female has fewer qualifications. A male provider can be seen in the case of minor problems not related to reproductive health (Iqbal 1995).

Lack of female doctors in private clinics and government hospitals was another problem. Two-thirds of the girls [in a predominantly Muslim slum community outside Bombay] never went to a male doctor unless absolutely necessary. Their mothers would get prescriptions and medicines on their behalf by describing the symptoms to the doctors.

— S.A. Udipi and M.A. Varghese, SNDT Women's University, Bombay, India

The Muslim religious practice of *purdah* prevents male doctors in Bangladesh from being present during the delivery of a child. Despite grave danger to the health of a woman during labour, mothers will forbid their daughters from going to urban hospitals for delivery, "where violation of *purdah* [is] inevitable" (Islam 1989, p. 234).

Male doctors also refuse to see female clients under certain circumstances. In Central Nepal, women have problems obtaining care from male providers when they are menstruating because they are believed to be polluted and untouchable at this time (Niraula 1994). Likewise, in Bangladesh, because "[c]hildbirth pollution is the most severe pollution of all … and delivering the baby, cutting the cord and cleaning up the blood are considered to be the most disgusting of tasks" (Jeffery et al. 1988, p. 106), some male doctors prefer to not handle deliveries and leave these tasks to female traditional birth attendants (Rozario 1995).

In a qualitative study of barriers that prevent women from using formal health services in Bolivia, the women interviewed said that "it should be women who attend to us" (Chiarella 1994, p. 214). More than half of the women interviewed in a study conducted in Kenya also said they would prefer a woman because "she is my kind" and because it would be easier to share problems with a woman (Ndhlovu 1994). Unfortunately, security concerns, constraints on the mobility of women, and the importance of women living with their families frequently prevent the recruitment of female health workers.

In addition to the sex of the provider, a recent study conducted in Kenya found that the age and maturity of the provider was also important to women. Women may be discouraged from seeking services because the "providers are younger than themselves and they have no wish to show their nakedness to young providers" (Ndhlovu 1994, p. 19). Women preferred "mature women who are married and have had babies" because they were believed to be able to understand and sympathize better with "women problems."

Adolescent females and women [are unwilling] to undress for the predominantly male health workers. In Nigeria, women are unwilling to have, as women in northern Nigeria put it, "strange men gazing at their nakedness."

— Uche Amazigo, University of Nigeria, Nsukka, Nigeria

CULTURALLY SENSITIVE SERVICES

Health care for women must be culturally acceptable, otherwise women may underutilize existing health services. Two studies, one from Bolivia, and one from China, explored the reluctance of indigenous women to use formal western-based health services because aspects of the services contradicted cultural beliefs and practices (Chiarella 1994; Zhang 1994).

Chiarella (1994) used qualitative research techniques to explore some of the reasons why indigenous women in the rural area of Cochabamba,

Women of the Tropical Chapare, Bolivia, [rarely] used western-based health services because procedures contradicted with [cultural] beliefs of what constituted desired practices. In some cases, the traditional and western-based health systems complemented each other. In other cases, the systems were very different and in opposition, and this led to the underutilization of services.

— Giovanna Chiarella, Health Research, Advice and Education Center, Cochabamba, Bolivia

Bolivia, did not use the formal health-care system although there was an appropriate supply of services and health programs. The area is comprised of numerous migratory peoples descended from different ethnic groups, which include Quechua, Aymara, and Oriental.

The researchers discovered that there were many differences between the traditional and western systems in their practices and beliefs related to prenatal care, labour, and delivery. Indigenous women were reluctant to attend hospitals for deliveries because of drawbacks inherent in the modern health-care system. Indigenous women preferred to deliver their babies at home because they could take "maté" tea to help in labour, they could be attended by their relatives and husband, they could walk around, they could be wrapped up warmly and wear their own clothes, they were not shaved or cut, and they were able to deliver vertically, squatting on their haunches. At the western-based hospital, however, nothing could be consumed, they were attended by strangers, they could not walk around during labour, they were undressed and given a hospital gown, the hospital was cold, an episiotomy was mandatory, and they had to deliver horizontally in the gynecological position. Women also said that hospital practices were unacceptable because they were unable to swaddle themselves so that the *magre* would not rise (the *magre* is a mythical organ that is believed to form behind the naval during pregnancy and which might rise and cause death by asphyxiation).

The traditional system also has different notions about the importance of the placenta. Among these indigenous people in Bolivia, the placenta is viewed as a continuance of life. Once the placenta is expelled, it is supposed to be washed and buried in a shady spot. In the case of a boy, the placenta should be buried in a coca patch, and in the case of a girl, it should be buried in the kitchen. If this rite is not adhered to, it is believed that a number of problems could arise. For example, the child may become sick and die or may turn out to be irresponsible or alcoholic, and the mother may also become ill (Chiarella 1994). Women said that it was important to follow this ritual with the placenta because it made them feel secure. This detailed ritual with the placenta is in sharp contrast to the western system in which the placenta is merely discarded. Women in rural villages in Yunnan, China, were also reluctant to have a hospital delivery, primarily because they were afraid of losing the placenta (Zhang 1995).

According to the traditional culture and religion, the placenta is thought to be the protective saint of the fetus, and it must be buried in a safe place to ensure the healthy development of the newborn. Not surprisingly, many women risk deliveries at home to ensure that they will be able to obtain the placenta for proper burial. Some scholars have suggested that hospital delivery would be more acceptable to women in these areas if return of the placenta were guaranteed.

— Kaining Zhang, Kunming Medical College, Kunming, China

Medical and hospital practices should ensure that they are culturally acceptable to the people who are intended to use them. Health services should adapt their working methods to accommodate traditional practices that are not detrimental to women's health (Turmen and AbouZahr 1994). Because of the importance placed on the placenta in some cultures, a ceremony for couples to welcome the placenta from the hospital to their home could be encouraged (Zhang 1994).

Although cultural norms and values must be respected, at some point it may be necessary for the health sector to challenge beliefs and practices that are harmful to women's health. In rural Myanmar, for example, qualitative research discovered that some traditional customs surrounding pregnancy and prenatal care were perfectly healthy; whereas others were potentially harmful to women (Win May et al. 1995). Healthy cultural practices during pregnancy, such as not lifting heavy loads, eating plenty of fruit and vegetables, and not avoiding any foods during pregnancy, should be encouraged by health providers. Other beliefs, such as the perception that edema is a normal phenomenon and that prenatal care is unnecessary if the mother is healthy, could be detrimental to pregnant women and should be discouraged.

Health personnel [in rural Myanmar] should educate pregnant mothers to be more aware of edema as a danger sign and to value and to use antenatal health-care services regularly. In this way, maternal mortality and morbidity could be reduced, and the health of the mother and child improved.

— Daw Win May, Institute of Nursing, Yangon, Myanmar

POOR QUALITY OF CARE

Women's decisions to seek care are influenced by their judgements about the nature and quality of health services. If women lack confidence in the available services, they generally do not use them. Women are often reluctant to use local health services because they believe, often correctly, that these services are poor. As a result, tertiary-level facilities are often seriously overcrowded because women consider them to be more effective and seek them out, despite the distances (AbouZahr 1994).

Many women have had poor personal experiences with health services, and their health is compromised by their reluctance to return to such services. According to one woman: "They treated me so bad, so bad, that I didn't say anything, I came back home and never went back" (Bonino 1994, p. 203). Another woman in the same study said: "The students were there, they undressed me, they all touched me. I am scared to go back" (p. 202). Women may not go for check-ups because the doctor "checks them up, and puts his finger in [the vagina]" (p. 202).

Women's health-seeking behaviour is also influenced by negative stories relayed to them by relatives and neighbours about the care they received: "My sister told me that they were going to cut me up from top to bottom — and so I never went" (Bonino 1994, p. 202). A study conducted in Malawi found that a significant percentage of women delivered their children at home because of negative past experiences or because others told them that midwives and staff had poor attitudes or were very unkind to women during labour (Lule and Ssembatya 1995). Women with positive attitudes to the staff at the health centre were almost three times more likely to deliver their children with the assistance of a trained person compared with those with negative attitudes. Some women said older female relatives advised them not to go to health centres or traditional birth attendants for delivery. Certain sources of information, such as friends and relatives, can be particularly credible to women who were making health-related decisions.

Judith Bruce (1990) of the Population Council in New York identified a number of quality of care elements that are important to women. These included the opportunity to make an informed choice, the provision of high-quality information, technical competence, good interpersonal relations,[21] follow-up and continuity mechanisms, and the appropriate constellation of services. However, results from numerous research studies have indicated that women in developing countries often receive very poor quality of care (WHO 1995). Haaland (1994), for example, reports that

> Rural women in Africa often have many complaints about the care they receive from health workers in their communities. They frequently accuse them of being impatient, rude, and careless. They also complain that health-care workers charge exorbitant prices for medicines and services. As a result of these problems, rural women to a large extent care for their health problems at home.

Women commonly complain that they are not provided with sufficient information. For example, women in rural Bolivia said they were dissatisfied because they were "poked everywhere" and the doctors "looked at us all over," but the doctors did not provide any explanations to the women (Chiarella 1994, p. 213). In a study conducted in Barbados and Grenada (Rodney 1995), health professionals felt that women did not need, or would not understand, their conditions, and therefore they neglected to communicate relevant, user-friendly, and sensitive information to them. When information **is** provided, health-education messages may not be provided in a way that is useful or easily understood by rural women — for example, written messages are of little use to women with low literacy levels.

Discussions from behind the screen were heard clearly by all strangers in the room, as was information relevant to the care of breasts and nipples, to personal hygiene, and to vaginal discharges and sexual activities.

— Ra'eda Al-Qutob, United Nations Fund for Population Activities (UNFPA)/WHO, Amman, Jordan, and Salah Mawajdeh, Jordan University of Science and Technology, Irbid, Jordan

It is generally believed that female clients place great emphasis on interpersonal relationships. Research findings, however, have highlighted a general lack of sensitivity on the part of providers in their dealings with

---

[21] Which would involve such qualities as privacy, respectful and responsive behaviour, being treated as an equal, and adequate time with the provider.

> The doctor should not scold one for taking the child [who is]
> dirty because if she goes for an emergency, she's not going to
> be thinking that she should wash him beforehand.
>
> — Quoted by Maria Bonino, Faculty of Medicine, Universidad de la República,
> Montevideo, Uruguay

clients. For example, women who received family-planning services in Kenya complained of long waiting times and said that they were not properly welcomed or made to feel comfortable by providers (Ndhlovu 1994). Mawajdeh et al. (1995) reported that many women in their study of the quality of prenatal care in Irbid, Jordan, were annoyed by the lack of auditory and visual privacy.

Women have also reported being harshly judged or scolded by health professionals because their lifestyle and behaviours were deemed to be inappropriate. One woman reported that her "sister was three months pregnant and when the doctor went out to call her she was smoking and she got scolded. And right then and there she did not go in" (Bonino 1994, pp. 202–203). Some women said they felt concerned about their level of cleanliness and type of dress, and they believed that it would be too much effort to "get ready" to go to the clinic. Women have been verbally abused by nurses and told that their clothes smelled (Bello 1995). Nomadic women in Illorin, Nigeria, reported that staff at the health facility (who were from another tribe) insulted them and told them that they behaved like the cows they herded (Bello 1995, p. 30). A woman in Iqbal's (1995) study reported that "they insulted me, and it couldn't go on like this; so I decided to stay at home."

Poor and otherwise marginalized women often feel they are treated differently than middle-class and paying clients. At a hospital in Bangladesh, Rozario (1995, p. 104) was told that "if a patient's guardians pay a large sum of money to the doctors and the nurses, they usually keep an eye on the patient. Otherwise, there is no guarantee that the patient is going to be attended to when needed. Mawajdeh et al. (1995) found that women who looked better received better communication and information from the clinic. A lower caste woman from a hill village in central Nepal (quoted in Niraula 1994, p. 157) reported the follwing:

> There is differential treatment in the health centre. If someone higher-caste and influential goes for treatment, he or she not only receives most of the time of the health post staff, but also receives free medicine. As for us, the poor, they direct us to buy from the shop .... When a family planning or health worker comes to the village, he never comes directly to us. He or she finds difficulty even to speak to us.

In many cases, there is a gulf between the worldview of the female client and that of the provider. The vast differences between clients and providers may act as a barrier to seeking care, and, if care is sought, may dramatically affect communication, understanding, and trust between the client and the provider.[22]

In a recent study of client-provider interactions, Simmons and Elias (1994, p. 4) state:

> Clients often experience providers as powerful individuals, who by social background and training are far removed from their own daily realities and concerns. Clients and providers bring very different expectations to their encounters, and these differences in perspective and power profoundly affect the nature of the interaction.

For example, one researcher described the difficulties in communication that developed between a client and provider at a regional hospital in the Eastern Province of South Africa[22] — the client was from a poor, rural, Xhosa family living in a remote area with little infrastructure. She spoke only Xhosa and adhered to a traditional way of life. In contrast, the medical practitioners consulted were white, male, English-speaking South Africans trained in medical schools and working in a regional hospital.

Women living in rural areas are disadvantaged. The viewpoints of urban-educated health workers and physicians, with their theories on anatomy and physiology and disease and treatment, are often very different than the viewpoints of rural women. This gap can present a barrier to the use of health services.

— S.A. Udipi and M.A. Varghese, SNDT Women's University, Bombay, India

Likewise, in central Nepal, where the service provider is usually a high-caste, educated, urban male and the patient is a lower-caste illiterate, poor, rural female, the status differences between the service providers and users "creates communication gaps and shadows the objectivity of the service" (Niraula 1994, p. 163).

Health workers who are from the same community as the people being served may have better success and provide better care than those from outside the community because they share a common cultural background and

---

[22] See Vincent, P.S., "The snake that broke Sitandile's neck." Unpublished paper submitted to the 1994–95 TDR/IDRC competition.

common experiences (Bonino 1994; Lange et al. 1994). Likewise, those who totally immerse themselves in a community may gain the trust and respect of the people being served — crucial elements to good health care. For example, a woman, when discussing a family doctor who had been working for years in her area, reported that, "with him it's different, he explains everything and you understand it all; it's as if he was one of us, as if he belonged here" (Bonino 1994, p. 203).

Good interpersonal care requires sufficient time on the part of the provider. Many physicians, however, reportedly do not provide enough time to let women talk about how or what they feel (AbouZahr 1994; Vlassoff 1994). Women should have the opportunity to discuss various psychosocial factors related to their health and well-being. In this way, they can learn about the relationship between the illness and disease and their lives as women, workers, mothers, and wives (Gupte 1994). However, doctors are often "too busy and therefore in too much of a hurry to finish each case and go to the next" (Ndhlovu 1994, p. 14).

School curricula, including medical and health education curricula, must address gender issues and the specific health needs of women. The basic training and refresher training courses of all health providers need reorientation to place health in the context of unequal gender status, and to provide women's perspectives on their needs and experiences.

— Boungnong Boupha, Lao Women's Union, Laos (see Boupha 1995)

Women are frustrated and discouraged when they travel great distances to the health centre by foot only to discover that the health worker is not there or that there is only one person available who has to treat many, and is therefore unable to provide adequate service and attention to individual clients (Chiarella 1994). Time of access for clients at some health facilities may be limited to only a fraction of the official 8 hours. Because health-care providers often receive little compensation for their work in public clinics, they may spend part of the working day at a private clinic to make extra money.

Providers in developing countries usually face numerous constraints that affect the quality of care they are able to provide. They tend to be overworked and underpaid, and health centres are invariably understaffed and underfinanced. As a result, they complain of having neither the time nor the energy to provide long explanations and high-quality care to their clients (Vlassoff 1994).

Health systems face other problems such as inadequate facilities, deficient professional training, poor renumeration for health professionals, and lack of social commitment.

— Constanza Collazos V., Centro de Investigaciones Multidisciplinarias en Desarrollo, Cali, Colombia

Ensuring the availability of essential supplies, equipment, and medication is a necessary requirement for good quality health care. However, there are often serious deficiencies in this domain (AbouZahr 1994; Atai-Okei 1994; Lwhiula 1994; Ren et al. 1995). Researchers from Africa, Asia, and Latin America have reported problems with condom availability, particularly in remote areas. A lack of gloves, disinfectant, and clean water has been reported in some family-planning services in Kenya: "cases have been cited ... where clients were seen crying because an IUD could not be removed because there was either no water or sterilizing lotion" (Ndhlovu 1994, p. 24).

The lack of integration of health services is another key factor that influences women's health-seeking behaviour and the quality of care received. In many countries, different types of health services (such as prenatal care, family planning, immunizations) are not integrated, and they may even be offered on different days (World Bank 1993). Women are therefore forced to return repeatedly to a clinic to receive care for their various health needs as well as the needs of their children. Given the heavy workloads and limited personal time available to women, strategies aimed at combining several health services at convenient times to meet women's needs should to be fully explored (World Bank 1993; Manderson 1994). When women present their children for care, it is an ideal opportunity to provide women themselves with other health services. Women would be more inclined to seek

Further away from the city, as one approaches the periphery, the facilities and support services dwindle. Communication becomes difficult and most things have to be done manually. This results in the feeling of being overburdened, which causes health workers' positive attitudes to slacken. Services become superficial.

— Daisy Tin Tin Saw, Cambodian Child Health Project, World Vision International, Phnom Penh, Cambodia

care for themselves when they present for care for their children rather than to arrange separate visits. The integration of efforts to prevent and treat STDs and HIV with general health-care services may also increase the chance that women will receive care for these stigmatizing diseases.

PREFERENCE FOR TRADITIONAL PRACTICES

The numerous barriers that prevent women from gaining access to health services, in addition to the poor quality of care sometimes delivered, may make traditional systems of medicine look more attractive than formal health services. Prohibitive costs associated with health services and the lack of time to travel to centres are two reasons why women prefer local traditional healers.

As a woman from the Benighat area of central Nepal (quoted in Niraula 1994, p. 163) said:

> Whenever I have [a headache], I visit the *dhami dai* (shaman brother). He chants some *mantra* touching my head three times and I feel much better after some time. *Dhami dai* is just across the house and I do not pay him anything for his services. If I go to the health post, it takes time and money. Where on earth am I going to get that much money for my illness? I get satisfaction from the services from him.

Rural women in Bangladesh reportedly preferred traditional birth attendants (*dai*) over doctors for the delivery of their children because they do not have to be concerned about their modesty in front of the female village *dai* who are from the area and familiar to them. Secondly, doctors are expensive, but "[a] *dai* is merely given a sari, if anything, and maybe a meal of chicken curry" (Rozario 1995). Traditional healers are also preferred by some women because they provide meaningful explanations of illness, in comparison with the limited information provided by modern health providers (Vlassoff 1994).

Chapter 8

New and Emerging Themes

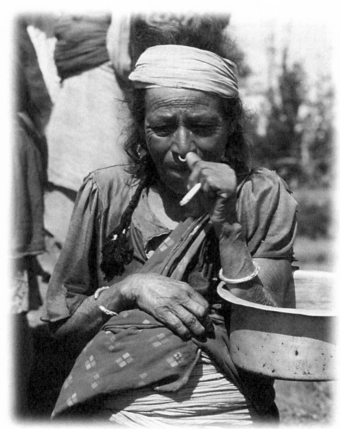

The health of women must be seen in the context of global changes and emerging trends in the world today. These changes are occurring rapidly, and their effects are being felt in the most isolated parts of the globe. Human health is, and will continue to be, profoundly affected during this continual and accelerating process of change.

— A. El Bindari Hammand, Global Commission on Women's Health, WHO, Geneva, Switzerland

The research areas that have been discussed — AIDS, the working environment, tropical diseases, and barriers to quality health care — are only a sample of the areas that urgently require more research from a gender perspective. During the regional workshops that formed the basis of this publication, six more priority research themes that have, until now, received relatively little attention from researchers and policymakers were identified: the health of older women, the health of girls during childhood and adolescence, mental health, women and tobacco, the effects of war on health, and violence against women. Although a thorough examination of these topics is beyond the scope of this book, they are briefly described.

HEALTH OF OLDER WOMEN

More research is needed on the health issues that affect older women. There has been close scrutiny of women's health related to reproduction, but the rest of women's lifespan has been largely ignored. Very little is know about the causes of morbidity and mortality in women over 45 years of age. Although women live longer than men in most societies, they do not necessarily live better. Many elderly women suffer from poor nutrition, reproductive ill-health, violence, alienation, loneliness, lifestyle-related diseases, and chronic and degenerative diseases.

The well-being of the growing aging population has health implications for the next generation of women. Females traditionally are the caregivers. As the population ages, the carers will eventually need care themselves — "who will care for the carers in their later years?" In the absence of government assistance, this responsibility tends to fall on the shoulders of daughters more often than sons. This represents yet another obligation assumed by women and added to their busy lives.

HEALTH OF ADOLESCENT GIRLS

Research also needs to focus specifically on the health of girls during child-hood and adolescence, times in women's lives when their health status in future years is often determined. Girls who are fed and nurtured less, given minimal access to health services and education, and denied the skills required for economic autonomy suffer the effects of this devaluation for the rest of their lives. The cumulative effects of illnesses, deprivation, and mal-nutrition in childhood can lead to impaired intellectual development and ill health later in life. Learning disabilities, anemia, and obstetrical complica-tions, which entail significant social and economic costs, are the result. Tropical diseases and STDs, including AIDS, can have unique health implica-tions for young girls. Young girls can also suffer health consequences associ-ated with heavy work burdens, such as chronic back pain, distorted pelvis, spontaneous abortions, detrimental effects on unborn children, and disabil-ity in old age.

MENTAL HEALTH

In both the industrialized and developing world, mental health issues faced by women have been grossly neglected. There is a need for more work on depression, which is a widespread psychiatric illness that is consistently more prevalent among women than men. There is also a need for more research on gender differences in overall rates of psychological distress and in the prevalence of specific symptoms.

WOMEN AND TOBACCO

Tobacco use, a major cause of morbidity and mortality throughout the world, is associated with higher rates of lung cancer, cardiovascular disease, and a host of other health problems. There is also well-accepted evidence that smoking during pregnancy is associated with higher risks for the fetus and eventual child, including higher rates of spontaneous abortions and low birth weight. Individuals exposed to second-hand smoke in their homes or work-places may also suffer detrimental health effects.

There is a significant lack of data on women and tobacco in develop-ing countries. Although the rates of female tobacco use are relatively low in developing countries (2–10%) compared with industrialized countries (20–35%), there is evidence that smoking prevalence rates for women in developing countries are increasing. In addition, in some developing nations, the percentage of women smoking cigarettes (or using other forms of tobacco such as reverse chutta, pan, and bidis) is already relatively high (for example, in Brazil, Chile, India, Nepal, and Papua New Guinea).

Concern has been expressed that the tobacco industry has identified women in the developing world as a huge potential market and is systematically targeting these women by exploiting ideas of independence, power, beauty, and emancipation to sell their products. As well, more women may soon take up smoking because it is rapidly becoming a new status symbol in the developing world. More research attention should be placed on women and tobacco in the developing world, and strategies to prevent increased tobacco use among women should be given full attention.

EFFECTS OF WAR ON HEALTH

In Asia, the effects of war continue to influence the health of women and men, particularly in Cambodia, Laos, and Viet Nam. Cambodia, for example, is one of the most densely mined countries in the world. Men continue to be maimed or killed by bombs and mines left in the fields and villages. Women are left with the additional responsibility of looking after these victims of war as well as their fatherless families. In addition, women have to face the acute social and environmental consequences of war because of their capacity as resource managers and providers for their families. The effects of these conditions on women's health should be addressed.

Research is also needed to explore the psychological effects of war. Over the last two decades, women in Cambodia, for example, have witnessed the execution of their husbands, watched loved ones die of starvation, or were raped and tortured. These horrific experiences have left psychological scars in the form of depression and post-traumatic-stress syndrome. More research attention should be placed on these health issues.

The negative health impact of forced migration also needs urgent attention. Current estimates of the number of refugees, immigrants, and displaced persons worldwide range from 40 to 100 million people. Because they live in unhygienic surroundings with few health resources, these individuals are prey to numerous health problems including cholera, malaria, chronic diarrhea, and AIDS. Crowded living conditions, combined with unemployment and lack of education, also foster addictions, sexual and physical abuse, depression, anxiety, and posttraumatic stress syndrome. According to the United Nations High Commissioner for Refugees (UNHCR), repeated and often brutal rapes are a common dimension of women's refugee experience.

VIOLENCE AGAINST WOMEN

Violence against women, a major public-health issue, is reaching alarming proportions in both developing and industrialized countries. Domestic violence and rape, for example, are significant causes of female morbidity and mortality. Assaults on women by their husbands or male partners are the world's most common form ·of violence. Surveys in recent years have indicated that about a quarter of the world's women are violently abused in their own homes, and community-based surveys have yielded even higher figures. Violence against women leads to psychological trauma, depression, substance abuse, injuries, STDs and HIV infection, and suicide. There is an urgent need for more research on violence against women in developing nations.

Chapter 9

Priorities for
Future Research

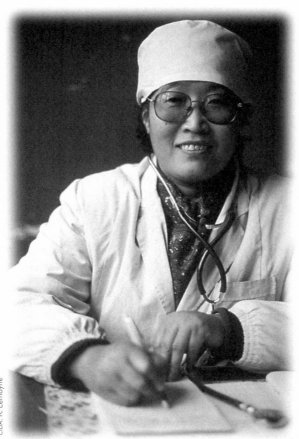

CIDA: R. Lemoyne

> *Now that we know more about women than ever before, and have identified the major problems they face, what can we do to accelerate actions which we know will alleviate unnecessary suffering and death? Among the large number of areas that need to be addressed, how can we choose the critical few that will make the greatest difference in the lives and health of many? How can we effectively involve women themselves in this process?*
>
> — A. El Bindari Hammand, Global Commission on Women's Health, WHO, Geneva, Switzerland

One of the objectives of the four IDRC-sponsored workshops on gender, health, and sustainable development was to translate the insights shared by participants into recommendations for future research to promote health and welfare for all. There is a definite need for further interdisciplinary research on various aspects of women's health. This research must fully integrate a gender perspective into the research protocol as it is conceived, carried out, analyzed, and disseminated. The dearth of health research that incorporates a gender perspective hinders the ability of decision-makers to design, plan, monitor, and evaluate effective women's health policies and programs.

Although each region faces unique concerns, common issues and problems clearly emerge. Researchers and organizations from around the world can achieve significant advancements in research on women's health by working cooperatively to consolidate experiences and results. It is hoped that this publication will inspire more collaborative work and networking among researchers working in the biomedical and social science fields.

Several priority research questions need to be explored in health studies. These questions should be tailored to the particular community or communities being studied, and the health implications of these questions should be explored. Key research questions have been divided into seven categories that broadly correspond to the chapters in this book: general issues, nutrition, education, AIDS, the working environment, tropical diseases, and barriers to quality health care. Many of these questions have been discussed in their respective chapters.

GENERAL ISSUES

✦ What are women's priority health concerns? What importance do women give to nonreproductive health issues? For example, how are tropical diseases and health issues associated with women's work perceived by women?

✦ How can the perspectives of women be incorporated into all stages of research, as well as interventions? How can women's viewpoints be fully integrated into the decision-making process in health policy?

✦ To what extent do policies and programs undertaken outside the health sector, aimed at improving the quality of women's lives (such as savings and credit programs and literacy courses), also lead to health improvements for women?

✦ What programs and policies will help to discourage harmful attitudes and practices against women, including son preference, female genital mutilation, violence, and discrimination against girls and women in educational opportunities and food allocation?

✦ What measures can be taken to empower women with regard to their own health? Would the formation of women's groups, where women can come together and talk openly about their problems, lead to increased self-esteem and to greater confidence to take control of their health and well-being?

✦ What obstacles hinder the adoption of a gender perspective in health research, and how can the obstacles be overcome?

✦ What strategies might help increase the number of female biomedical and social scientists working in women's health?

EDUCATION

✦ What educational opportunities do women and men, girls and boys, receive? How does the community or communities being studied view the education of girls? How does poverty of education affect women's health and well-being?

✦ To what extent does a woman's level of education influence her decision-making power on health-related matters within the family and the community?

✦ What are the links between women's education and opportunities in the work force? What types of subjects are women and men encouraged to study?

✦ How can families and communities be encouraged to place more emphasis on the education of girls?

NUTRITION

✦ Is there any difference between the nutritional intake of girls and boys, women and men? Who eats first and last? Who eats the most and least?

✦ What factors affect gender-differentiated nutritional levels? How can the discrimination against women's access to food that exists in some societies be overcome?

✦ Who decides on what crops to cultivate, who farms them, and who gets the money for the produce?

✦ Do women suffer from specific health problems, such as fatigue, night blindness, bone deformities, and stunting, that result from nutritional deficiencies?

✦ Who decides how much money is to be spent on food and what sorts of foods should be bought?

✦ Who prepares the food? What is the health status of the family member who prepares the food?

✦ What factors lead to the high rate of nutrition-related diseases among Caribbean women and how can they be overcome?

✦ How does environmental degradation affect family nutritional levels? Where environmental degradation makes it difficult to obtain adequate food, does this have a greater impact on women, as family food providers?

AIDS

✦ To what extent do women and men suffer from AIDS?

✦ Is there a physiological basis to the susceptibility of HIV infection in women, particularly among young women and postmenopausal women?

✦ What factors increase the risk of HIV infection among young women (pressures to be sexually active at an early age, sexual relations with older men, lack of decision-making power)? What strategies could be used to delay the entry of females into sexual activity? How can young women gain greater control over how, when, and with whom they have sexual intercourse?

✦ Will effective education programs tailored to adolescents girls and boys, both in and out of school, on a wide range of sexual and reproductive health issues, including STD and HIV prevention, lead to a decrease in STD and HIV infection rates among adolescents? How can the restrictions that in some societies prevent adolescents, particularly young women, from access to information on sexuality, contraception, and disease prevention be overcome?

✦ Why do women with AIDS have a poorer prognosis than men? Is this related to biological differences? What role do other factors play (later diagnosis for women, less access to health services, lack of social support, and poor knowledge of early HIV symptoms)?

✦ What strategies might increase the diagnosis and treatment of STDs in women and men? How can the shame, embarrassment, and stigma associated with STDs, especially among women, be challenged? If STD services were offered in private consultations in conjunction with primary health care and family-planning services, would this increase the chances of women reporting for STDs? Would screening for asymptomatic STD infections in women in family-planning clinics lead to increased diagnosis? Would the inclusion of high quality, gender-sensitive instruction on STDs in the professional training of health providers lead to greater diagnosis of STDs among women?

✦ How do women and men believe that a HIV infection is acquired? How can misperceptions about HIV and AIDS be effectively clarified? (For example, women and men need to be informed that married men or those in steady relationships can expose their partners to HIV and that monogamous women can be at risk; that some men are bisexual and can expose their partners to HIV risk; that AIDS is not restricted to homosexuals, prostitutes, and drug users; that an HIV-infected individual can look "healthy"; and that there is a latency period of about 6 months between the time of infection and a positive HIV test).

✦ Are women able to ask their partners to use condoms? Who decides whether or not to use condoms? How do women and men feel about condoms? Are condoms widely available?

✦ How can women be empowered to take control of their bodies? Would assertiveness-training programs and initiatives aimed at building women's self-esteem improve women's ability to determine the conditions under which sexual intercourse occurs? Can group counseling help women deal with these issues?

✦ If community women were trained in AIDS-prevention measures and encouraged to visit their neighbours to discuss these issues face-to-face, would this be an effective AIDS-prevention strategy?

✦ Would the creation of an HIV-prevention method that women could control (that would not require partner awareness, compliance, or action) lead to decreased HIV transmission to women?

✦ Does a desire for children influence condom use? Would women and men be more likely to use an HIV-prevention method that would let sperm pass unharmed (and therefore permit conception)?

✦ What policies and programs can be designed and implemented to encourage men to take greater responsibility for AIDS prevention? How can condoms be made more acceptable to men? Would the use of male workers in condom distribution campaigns lead to greater male acceptance of condoms?

✦ How can strategies for AIDS education be tailored to the needs poor women, women with low literacy levels, and women from different cultural backgrounds? Do radio and newspaper messages effectively reach women? Are creative educational approaches (such as packaging prevention messages in soap operas and community dramas) effective?

✦ How can communication barriers between women and men on matters related to sexuality be reduced? How can women and men be motivated to openly discuss extramarital sex, the risks of contracting STDs, and the need for condom use?

✦ How are women and men who are living with AIDS treated by their families and the community at large?

✦ How can the legal and customary inheritance practices in some societies be changed to allow women the right of ownership to their husbands' property when he dies?

✦ To what extent do women and men turn to prostitution as a source of income?

✦ Are certain women in society more likely to get STDs (and AIDS) than others? To what extent do race and class variables intersect with gender?

✦ Would an increase in the economic autonomy of women — by, for example, changing laws that perpetuate women's economic dependence on men by denying them the right to independent property ownership or tenancy, or prohibiting access to certain forms of employment or financial credit — lead to an increase in the ability of women to demand safer sex?

✦ How can harmful cultural practices that increase HIV risk for women and generally endanger women's health (such as female genital mutilation and vaginal drying) be stopped?

✦ To what extent are women and men encouraged by society to engage in extramarital sex? How can traditional practices and rituals in which women and men are permitted to have extramarital sexual contact (which carries the risk of STD transmission) be challenged?

✦ Are women and men exposed to sexual violence? Would enforced laws against rape and sexual violence decrease the incidence of sexual violence against women as well as the risk of AIDS?

✦ Would messages targeted and tailored to male bisexuals and their partners lead to a decreased risk of AIDS among women?

THE WORKING ENVIRONMENT

✦ What constitutes women's work and men's work? How do the differentiated life spaces of women and men and their gender-determined roles and responsibilities affect their health? Who works at a fast pace? Who experiences sexual harassment? Who handles heavy weights? Who works in positions of authority and decision-making? Who works on assembly lines? Who works shift work? Who has repetitive and monotonous work? Who performs rapid and repetitive hand movements?

✦ What measures can be taken to ensure that women's "invisible work" is properly measured and that the health risks associated with women's work in the informal sector are properly addressed?

✦ What are the potential health risks associated with women's agricultural work? What are the health risks to women from excessive pesticide use?

✦ What policies and programs will help ensure that women are properly informed of the ill-effects associated with agrochemicals and provided with protective clothing and masks?

✦ Would improvements in the general status of women's health and well-being (such as better nutrition and more rest) improve their ability to cope with detrimental health conditions associated with the workplace?

✦ What are the psychological health effects associated with the common characteristics of women's work (monotonous, repetitive tasks, a lack of control over the external environment, little opportunity for communication with others, and minimal decision-making and creativity)?

✦ How can increased recognition be achieved for women's role as health providers within the formal health-care system? How do we ensure that female health providers are not exploited and that their work is fully recognized? How can the working conditions of female health workers be improved?

✦ What are the health hazards associated with women's work in the industrial sector of developing nations, particularly in the rapidly expanding free-trade and export-producing zones? How do the forces of globalization and increased international trade affect the working conditions and health standards of female workers in developing nations? How can these forces best be dealt with?

✦ What is a woman's daily activity pattern? Who cares for children when they are sick? Who ensures the provision of safe and abundant water? Who obtains fuel and prepares the food? Who maintains the kitchen garden? To what extent do the competing demands placed on women (paid work outside the home and childrearing and household management) create physical and mental stress?

✦ What measures and technologies might serve to lessen the daily burden of women's domestic responsibilities (perhaps water pumps for people of shorter physical stature)? How can other family members be encouraged to support women with their childcare and household responsibilities?

✦ What are the working conditions and specific health concerns of home-workers?

✦ What are the health implications of carrying water over long distances in heavy containers for many years? To what extent are women and men exposed to indoor air pollution, and how does this affect health? How can these health risks be minimized?

✦ To what extent can modifications to home cooking and heating facilities — such as stove design, ventilation design, and fuel type — reduce women's exposure to the detrimental effects of indoor air pollution?

✦ Do the effects of environmental degradation have similar consequences on the health and livelihoods of women and men?

✦ What are women's hours of work and leisure compared with those of men? How does minimal discretionary time affect health?

✦ How is women's work valued, compared with men's work? What are women's income levels compared with men's? What types of activities do women and men perform without financial compensation? To what extent do wage levels influence the health status of women and men?

✦ What factors compound or mitigate poverty and poor health within female-headed households?

✦ What steps can be taken to ensure that adequate occupational health and safety standards, and enforcement measures, are put into place with regard to the risks associated with women's work? What strategies will ensure that protective legislation is not used to justify discriminatory labour practices and keep women out of better paying jobs? How can we ensure that other legislation aimed at protecting women (such as maternity-leave benefits) does not end up depressing their wages or discouraging their employment?

✦ To what extent are women's jobs, compared with men's, supported by unions? What percentage of union representatives are women and men? How can the representation of women in trade unions be increased? How can union representatives be encouraged to make the health concerns of women a priority?

✦ Do women and men work within a contractual situation? Is their work covered by health and social-security protection? In the case of a work-related illness, who pays for medical care? Can medical leave be taken?

✦ What steps can be taken to effectively extend the protection of labour and social security laws to part-time, temporary jobs and seasonal and homebased workers?

✦ How can we ensure that workers are properly educated about the hazards associated with their work?

✦ To what extent can organizations of women workers play a role in pressuring for better wages and working conditions and reducing occupational risks?

TROPICAL DISEASES

✦ What is the effect of sex on the susceptibility and intensity of infection and progression of disease? How do factors such as pregnancy, the generally poor nutritional status of women, and intercurrent infections influence disease susceptibility in women?

✦ To what extent do women's and men's gender-differentiated "life spaces" influence their exposure to tropical diseases? What sociocultural factors (such as clothing patterns and religious practices) predispose women and men to tropical diseases and what practices safeguard women and men? Would the mapping of women's and men's culturally prescribed and gender-differentiated responsibilities and activities lead to more effective interventions to prevent and control tropical diseases among women and men?

✦ Are women living in poorer socioeconomic conditions (such as with poor housing and lack of adequate hygiene practices) disproportionately affected by tropical diseases?

✦ How are women and men differentially affected by the stigmatizing effect of tropical diseases? What are the social and psychological effects (anxiety and depression) of disfigurement for women? What are the implications for women and men when diseases are believed to be sexually transmitted? How can health services be made more aware of the stigmas associated with the disfigurement and disability that result from some tropical diseases, especially for women?

✦ To what extent do women have access to diagnosis and treatment for tropical diseases? Are personnel and facilities for the detection, documentation, and treatment of tropical diseases available for women who attend health-care clinics?

✦ What is the impact on women when other family members are ill? To what extent do women feel they are the sole or principal caretakers of the family? Who diagnoses family illnesses? Who cares for the sick? Who accompanies sick family members to the health centre? How can men be encouraged to take more responsibility for caring for the sick?

✦ What sort of support and resources should be provided for those involved formally or informally in the care of sick and dying individuals?

✦ To what extent does a woman's illness impact on other family members? What are the effects of a woman's illness on children, for example, its effects on absenteeism, drop-out rates, and learning outcomes of school-age girls?

✦ Who is responsible for assuring that disease-control interventions are carried out? For example, who is responsible for reimpregnating bednets every 6 months? Who is responsible for maintaining household sanitation practices?

✦ Because the ultimate success and effectiveness of interventions may depend on the participation of women, what steps can be taken to ensure that women are involved in disease-control interventions? At the same time, what strategies might lead to a more equitable distribution of family roles? How can health interventions be designed to eliminate gender bias and to take into account the disproportionate demands that child-rearing, household duties, and income-generating activities make on women's time? Would the targeting of messages about family health to both women and men, rather than solely to women (which perpetuates the idea that family health is primarily or exclusively the responsibility of women) be helpful? How can men be encouraged to take a more active role in creating and maintaining a healthy home environment, rather than leaving the entire responsibility to women?

✦ Do women and men properly understand the causes, symptoms, transmission routes, and prevention and treatment strategies for tropical diseases?

✦ What role do men and other family members play in decision-making about health-related practices?

✦ To what extent do health interventions targeted at women lead to changes in health-related practices and beliefs among other family members?

✦ How do we ensure that the considerable health-related knowledge and expertise of women, which is related to their role as health providers in the formal health-care sector and in the community and home, is fully acknowledged? If women, the major users of health services, were consulted during the conceptualization of health-care policies and programs, would this lead to health gains for women and men?

BARRIERS TO QUALITY HEALTH CARE

✦ What factors prevent women from knowing and understanding their bodies? Can women openly discuss health issues? Would greater education on health-related matters increase the ability of women to recognize the signs and symptoms of illness? How can cultural restrictions and taboos that prevent women from understanding issues related to their reproductive and sexual health best be dealt with?

✦ What are women's time-use patterns for their health and personal needs? Given women's busy lives and the competing demands on their time, what strategies might make it easier for women to visit modern health services? Would it be helpful to change the hours when clinics are open (perhaps opening clinics in the evening) to accommodate women's work schedules? If health services were offered where women work, would this increase the opportunity for women to receive care?

204 ✦ THE HEALTH GAP

✦ What are the attitudes of society to women who are ill? Who looks after women when they are sick, and who accompanies them to health services? What do women feel that they can expect in terms of men's support? How can other family members be encouraged to help women with their tasks so women can have enough time to fully recover from illness?

✦ How do women prioritize health compared with other social, economic, environmental, and political concerns? How do women prioritize their health compared with the health of their children and other family members?

✦ What health problems do women consider to be serious and not serious? How many ailments exist among women and never receive medical assistance? How can we instill in women the importance of making their own health care a priority? Because women tend to place great importance on their children, would messages that emphasize the notion that women must take care of their health to maintain their child's health be persuasive? Would strategies aimed at improving women's self-esteem lead to their increased use of health services?

✦ Who are the significant others that participate in decision-making regarding women's access to health care? If women were encouraged to go to health centres when they were ill, would this improve the chance of them going? How can family members and the community at large be encouraged to support women's health?

✦ What are the stigmatizing diseases and conditions in the community? How can health services be more sensitive to the shame and embarrassment felt by women with regard to stigmatizing diseases and illnesses?

✦ What psychological barriers (such as depression, apathy, and fear) prevent women from accessing care and how can they be reduced?

✦ How far do people have to travel to reach a health centre? How can health services be made more physically accessible to women? Would mobile health clinics and the provision of transportation improve the accessibility of health services?

✦ What is the extent of women's physical mobility outside the home compared with men's? How can the cultural restrictions on women's mobility in some societies be overcome? If elderly widows of secure honour and status were trained as health workers to visit women in domestic seclusion, would this improve access to care for women whose mobility is restricted?

✦ How much, if anything, does it cost to use the health centre? Is there a cost associated with transportation to the health centre? What sorts of schemes of payment are suitable to women? What are women's means for the purchase of drugs? Which family member(s) decides whether the costs associated with health are worthwhile?

✦ Who are the health practitioners who provide care to the community or communities being studied? What is the sex of the health worker? Do women feel comfortable visiting this provider? What does the wider community think of the health worker and clinic? Is there a difference in quality of care if the provider belongs to the community being served?

✦ Would the availability of female providers increase the liklihood that women would go to modern health services? Given the reluctance of women to see male providers in some societies, how can more female providers, especially mature women, be recruited, particularly for sexual health issues?

✦ How can we ensure that health care for women is culturally acceptable? At the same time, what is the best way to challenge beliefs and practices that are harmful to women's health and well-being?

✦ To what extent would integrated services (such as tropical disease, family planning, reproductive health, and pediatric services) lead to improvements in the quality of care delivered to women? If health services for women were available when they presented their children for care, would this improve the chances of women seeking care for themselves?

✦ How can we ensure that women with low levels of education and lower socioeconomic positions receive high-quality information and counseling and care from providers?

✦ What sources of information (such as friends and relatives) are particularly credible to women when making health-related decisions?

✦ How can health-education messages be provided in a way that is useful and easily understood by rural women?

✦ What level of sensitivity to gender issues exists among health providers? Are providers knowledgeable about women's health concerns? Do providers treat women as persons in their own right, or as nurturers and the bearers of children?

✦ How can the quality of care provided to women be improved given the constraints faced by providers (such as overwork, low pay, and many clients)?

✦ What quality of care elements are important to women (for example, privacy, nonjudgemental attitudes, and sufficient time with provider)?

✦ Who do women consult for health care, at what stage of illness, and for what conditions? What type of health facilities do women consult first?

Why do women sometimes prefer traditional healers? What are the aspects of healers that make them attractive to women?

✦ What strategies could be used to improve interpersonal relationships between female patients and health providers?

✦ How and to what extent can training in interpersonal and communication skills, counseling, and the use of a gender perspective that emphasizes sensitive and respectful care lead to a change in the attitudes and behaviour of health-care providers?

Acronyms and Abbreviations

AIDS	acquired immune deficiency syndrome
ASA	acetylsalicylic acid
AZT	azidothymidine
ENGENDER	Centre for Environment, Gender and Development
FAO	Food and Agriculture Organization of the United Nations
HIV	human immunodeficiency virus
ICPD	International Conference on Population and Development
ICRW	International Centre for Research on Women
IDRC	International Development Research Centre
ILO	International Labour Organisation
IUD	intrauterine device
MEK	methyl ethyl ketone
NGO	nongovermental organization
SENA	Self-Employed Women's Association
STD	sexually transmitted disease
TCE	trichloroethylene
TDR	WHO Special Programme for Research and Training in Tropical Diseases
UNDP	United Nations Development Programme
UNFPA	United Nations Fund for Population Activities
UNHCR	United Nations High Commission for Refugees
WAND	Women and Development Unit, University of the West Indies
WHO	World Health Organization

Bibliography

Abegaz, Z.; Junge, B. 1990. Women's workloads and time use in four peasant associations in Ethiopia. United Nations Children's Fund, New York, NY, USA.

AbouZahr, C. 1994. Should all research on quality of care in women's health be intervention-related? Paper presented at the workshop on the quality of health care for women in developing countries, 15–17 October 1994, Budapest, Hungary. World Health Organization, Geneva, Switzerland. 6 pp.

Acevedo, D. 1994. Gender and occupational health in Venezuela. In Wijeyaratne, P.; Hatcher Roberts, J.; Kitts, J.; Jones Arsenault, L., ed., Gender, health, and sustainable development: a Latin American perspective. Proceedings of a workshop held in Montevideo, Uruguay, 26–29 April 1994. International Development Research Centre, Ottawa, ON, Canada. pp. 94–102.

Adeokun, L.A. 1994. Gender differentials and household issues in AIDS. In Wijeyaratne, P.; Jones Arsenault, L.; Hatcher Roberts, J.; Kitts, J., ed., Gender, health, and sustainable development: proceedings of a workshop held in Nairobi, Kenya, 5–8 October 1993. International Development Research Centre, Ottawa, ON, Canada. pp. 22–31.

Agarwal, B. 1986. Cold hearths and barren slopes — the woodfuel crisis in the Third World. The Riverdale Company, Riverdale, MD, USA. 209 pp.

Agyeman, D.K. 1992. Care of AIDS patients in Ghana. Paper presented at the SAREC workshop on AIDS and society, Kampala, Uganda, 15–16 December 1992. AIDS Control Program, Ministry of Health, Entebbe, Uganda.

Agyepong, I.A. 1992. Women and malaria: social, economic, cultural, and behavioural determinants of malaria. In Wijeyaratne, P.; Rathgeber, E.M.; St.-Onge, E., ed., Women and tropical diseases. International Development Research Centre, Ottawa, ON, Canada. pp. 176–193.

Ahikire, J. 1991. Worker struggles, the labour process, and the question of control: the case of United Garment Industry Limited. Centre for Basic Research, Kampala, Uganda. CBR Working Paper 16, 55 pp.

Airhihenbuwa, C.O.; DiClemente, R.J.; Wingood, G.M.; Lowe, A. 1992. HIV/AIDS education and prevention among African-Americans: a focus on culture. AIDS Education and Prevention, 4(3), 267–276.

Alilio, M.S. 1994. Gender and acceptance of technologies for tropical diseases: impregnated mosquito bednets for malaria control. In Wijeyaratne, P.; Jones Arsenault, L.; Hatcher Roberts, J.; Kitts, J., ed., Gender, health, and sustainable development: proceedings of a workshop held in Nairobi, Kenya, 5–8 October 1993. International Development Research Centre, Ottawa, ON, Canada. pp. 102–109.

Amazigo, U. 1994. Gender and tropical diseases in Nigeria: a neglected dimension. In Wijeyaratne, P.; Jones Arsenault, L.; Hatcher Roberts, J.; Kitts, J., ed., Gender, health, and sustainable development: proceedings of a workshop held in Nairobi, Kenya, 5–8 October 1993. International Development Research Centre, Ottawa, ON, Canada. pp. 85–99.

Anarfi, J.K. 1992. Coping strategies of households with AIDS sufferers in Ghana. Paper presented at the SAREC workshop on AIDS and society, Kampala, Uganda, 15–16 December 1992. AIDS Control Program, Ministry of Health, Entebbe, Uganda.

Ankrah, E. 1991. AIDS and the social side of health. Social Science and Medicine, 32(9), 967–980.

Anyangwe, S.; Njikam, O.; Kouemeni, L.; Awa, P.; Wansi, E. 1994. Gender issues in the control and prevention of malaria and urinary schistosomiasis in endemic foci in Cameroon. In Wijeyaratne, P.; Jones Arsenault, L.; Hatcher Roberts, J.; Kitts, J., ed., Gender, health, and sustainable development: proceedings of a workshop held in Nairobi, Kenya, 5–8 October 1993. International Development Research Centre, Ottawa, ON, Canada. pp. 77–84.

APDC (Asian and Pacific Development Centre). 1990. Asia and Pacific women's resource and action series: health. APDC, Kuala Lumpur, Malaysia. 298 pp.

———— 1992. Asian and Pacific women's resource and action series: environment. APDC, Kuala Lumpur, Malaysia. 237 pp.

Atai-Okei, H.R. 1994. Maternal and child health care in Teso, Uganda: social issues. In Wijeyaratne, P.; Jones Arsenault, L.; Hatcher Roberts, J.; Kitts, J., ed., Gender, health, and sustainable development: proceedings of a workshop held in Nairobi, Kenya, 5–8 October 1993. International Development Research Centre, Ottawa, ON, Canada. pp. 205–210.

Awofeso, N. 1992. Appraisal of the knowledge and attitude of Nigerian nurses toward leprosy. Leprosy Review, 63, 169.

Ayele, T. 1988. Current state of visceral leishmaniasis in Ethiopia. In Walton, B.C.; Wijeyaratne, P.; Modabber, R., ed., Research on control strategies for the leishmaniasis: proceedings of an international workshop held in Ottawa, Canada, 1–4 June 1987. International Development Research Centre, Ottawa, ON, Canada. IDRC-MR184e, 41–50.

Ayers, L.; Cusack, M.; Crosby, F. 1993. Combining work and home. Occupational Medicine: State of the Art Reviews, 8(4), 821–831.

Badaro, R. 1988. Current state in regard to leishmaniasis in Brazil. In Walton, B.C.; Wijeyaratne, P.; Modabber, R., ed., Research on control strategies for the leishmaniasis: proceedings of an international workshop held in Ottawa, Canada, 1–4 June 1987. International Development Research Centre, Ottawa, ON, Canada. IDRC-MR184e, 91–100.

Bailey, W.; Hardee, K; Smith, S; Villemski, M.; McDonald, O.; Clyde, M. 1995. Geographical and medical barriers to family planning services in rural Jamaica. In Hatcher Roberts, J.; Kitts, J.; Jones Arsenault, L., ed., Gender, health, and sustainable development: perspectives from Asia and the Caribbean. Proceedings of workshops held in Singapore, 23–26 January 1995, and in Bridgetown, Barbados, 6–9 December 1994. International Development Research Centre, Ottawa, ON, Canada. pp. 326–337.

Baldwin, J.I.; Whitely, S.; Balwin, J.D. 1990. Changing AIDS and fertility-related behaviour: the effectiveness of AIDS education. Journal of Sex Research, 27, 245–262.

Balmer, D. 1994. Gender, counselling and STDs/AIDS. *In* Wijeyaratne, P.; Jones Arsenault, L.; Hatcher Roberts, J.; Kitts, J., ed., Gender, health, and sustainable development: proceedings of a workshop held in Nairobi, Kenya, 5–8 October 1993. International Development Research Centre, Ottawa, ON, Canada. pp. 46–58.

Basnet Dixit, S. 1990. Hear no AIDS, see no AIDS, speak no AIDS. HIMAL, 3(3), 26–30.

Bassett, M.T.; Mhloyi, M. 1993. AIDS and sexually transmitted diseases: an important connection. *In* Berer, M.; Ray, S., ed., Women and HIV/AIDS: an international resource book. Pandora, London, UK.

Batliwala, S. 1988. Fields of rice — health hazards for women and unborn children. Manushi (New Delhi), 46, 31–35.

Bello, K. 1995. Vesicovaginal fistula (VVF): only to a woman accursed. *In* Hatcher Roberts, J.; Vlassoff, C., ed., The female client and the health-care provider. International Development Research Centre, Ottawa, ON, Canada. pp. 77–84.

Berer, M.; Ray, S., ed. 1993. Women and HIV/AIDS: an international resource book. Pandora, London, UK. 383 pp.

Bernardi, R.; Mouriño, P. 1991. Diseño y validación de un instrumento para valorar el entorno psicosocial. Salud Pública de México, 33(1).

Berr, X.D. 1994. Gender and occupational health in Chile. *In* Wijeyaratne, P.; Hatcher Roberts, J.; Kitts, J.A.; Jones Arsenault, L., ed., Gender, health, and sustainable development: a Latin American perspective. Proceedings of a workshop held in Montevideo, Uruguay, 26–29 April 1994. International Development Research Centre, Ottawa, ON, Canada. pp. 77–84.

Bhattacharyya, J.; Hati, A.K. 1995. The adverse effects of kala-azar (visceral leishmaniasis) in women. *In* Hatcher Roberts, J.; Vlassoff, C., ed., The female client and the health-care provider. International Development Research Centre, Ottawa, ON, Canada. pp. 43–63.

Binh, N.T.H. 1995. Current health status of women and children in Vietnam and the role of the Vietnam Women's Union. *In* Hatcher Roberts, J.; Kitts, J.; Jones Arsenault, L., ed., Gender, health, and sustainable development: perspectives from Asia and the Caribbean. Proceedings of workshops held in Singapore, 23–26 January 1995, and in Bridgetown, Barbados, 6–9 December 1994. International Development Research Centre, Ottawa, ON, Canada. pp. 17–21.

Bledsoe, C. 1990. The politics of AIDS, condoms, and heterosexual relations in Africa: recent evidence from the local print media. *In* Handwerker, W.P., ed., Births and power: social change and the politics of reproduction. Westview Press, Boulder, CO, USA.

Bonilla, E.; Kuratomi, L.S.; Rodriguez, P.; Rodriguez, A. 1991. Salud y desarrollo: aspectos socioeconomicos de la malaria en Colombia. Plaza and Janes, Bogotá, Colombia.

Bonino, M. 1994. Psychosocial determinants of the use of maternal-child health services in areas of poverty. *In* Wijeyaratne, P.; Hatcher Roberts, J.; Kitts, J.; Jones Arsenault, L., ed., Gender, health, and sustainable development: a Latin

American perspective. Proceedings of a workshop held in Montevideo, Uruguay, 26–29 April 1994. International Development Research Centre, Ottawa, ON, Canada. pp. 199–207.

Borges, A. 1993. Proyecto de investigación: salud reproductiva en trabajadoras de textiles. La Victoria, Aragua, Venezuela.

Boupha, B. 1995. Women's health activities towards health for all by the year 2000. In Hatcher Roberts, J.; Kitts, J.; Jones Arsenault, L., ed., Gender, health, and sustainable development: perspectives from Asia and the Caribbean. Proceedings of workshops held in Singapore, 23–26 January 1995, and in Bridgetown, Barbados, 6–9 December 1994. International Development Research Centre, Ottawa, ON, Canada. pp. 22–32.

Brabin, L.; Brabin, B.J. 1992. Parasitic infections in women and their consequences. Advances in Parasitology, 31, 1–81.

Breilh, J. 1994. Health at work: a gender perspective. In Wijeyaratne, P.; Hatcher Roberts, J.; Kitts, J.A.; Jones Arsenault, L., ed., Gender, health, and sustainable development: a Latin American perspective. Proceedings of a workshop held in Montevideo, Uruguay, 26–29 April 1994. International Development Research Centre, Ottawa, ON, Canada. pp. 85–93.

Brieger, W.R.; Watts, S.; Yacoob, M. 1989. Guinea worm, maternal morbidity and child health. Journal of Tropical Paediatrics, 35, 285–288.

Broadbent, E. 1995. Will next month's UN conference set back women's rights? Globe and Mail (Toronto), 10 August 1995, p. A19.

Bruce, J. 1990. Fundamental elements of the quality of care: a simple framework. Studies in Family Planning, 21(2), 61–91.

Burden, D.S.; Gottleib, N. 1987. Women's socialisation and feminist groups. In Brody C.M., ed., Women's therapy groups: paradigms of feminist treatment. Springer Publishing Co., New York, NY, USA. 260 pp.

Butler, I.; Pizurki, H.; Mejia, A. 1987. Women as providers of health care. World Health Organization, Geneva, Switzerland. 163 pp.

Bwayo, J. 1991. Long-distance truck drivers: knowledge and attitudes concerning sexually transmitted diseases and sexual behaviour. East African Medical Journal, 68, 715–719.

Byron, P. 1991. HIV: the national scandal. Ms., January–February 1991, pp. 24–29.

Caldwell, J.C. 1993. Health transition: the cultural, social and behavioural determinants of health in the Third World. Social Science and Medicine, 36(2), 125–135.

Campbell, C. 1990. Women and AIDS. Social Science and Medicine, 30(4), 407–415.

Canadian Institute of Child Health. 1994. The health of Canada's children (2nd ed.). Canadian Institute of Child Health, Ottawa, ON, Canada. 175 pp.

Caplan, P. 1987. The cultural construction of sexuality. Tavistock Publications, London, UK. 304 pp.

Carasco, J. 1994. Gender and health effects of environmental stress among Kampala textile workers. In Wijeyaratne, P.; Jones Arsenault, L.; Hatcher Roberts, J.; Kitts, J., ed., Gender, health, and sustainable development: proceedings of a workshop held in Nairobi, Kenya, 5–8 October 1993. International Development Research Centre, Ottawa, ON, Canada. pp. 137–147.

Cardaci, D. 1992. Mujeres, cuidado de la salud y violencia: mujer, salud y autocuidado — memorias. Pan American Health Organization, Washington, DC, USA.

Carovano, K. 1991. More than mothers and whores: redefining the AIDS-prevention needs of women. International Journal of Health Services, 21(1), 131–142.

Carpenter, C.; Mayer, K.; Stein, M.; Leibman, B.; Fisher, A.; Fiore, T. 1991. Human immunodeficiency virus infection in North American women: experience with 200 cases and a review of the literature. Medicine, 70(5), 307–325.

Carrier, J. 1989. Sexual behaviour and the spread of AIDS in Mexico. Medical Anthropology, 10, 129–142.

Chatterjee, M. 1990. Indian women: their health and economic productivity. World Bank, Washington, DC, USA. World Bank Discussion Paper 109, 130 pp.

Chauvin, L. 1993. Pink plague changes course. WorldAIDS, 26, 10.

Chavkin, W. 1984. Double exposure: women's health hazards on the job and at home. Monthly Review Press, New York, NY, USA. 276 pp.

Chen, L.C.; Huq, E.; Souza, D. 1981. Sex bias in the family allocation of food and health care in rural Bangladesh. Population and Development Review, 7(1), 55–70.

Chiarella, G. 1994. Knowledge, attitudes and practices of women concerning pregnancy and birth. In Wijeyaratne, P.; Hatcher Roberts, J.; Kitts, J.A.; Jones Arsenault, L., ed., Gender, health, and sustainable development: a Latin American perspective. Proceedings of a workshop held in Montevideo, Uruguay, 26–29 April 1994. International Development Research Centre, Ottawa, ON, Canada. pp. 208–219.

Cochran, S.D.; Peplau, L.A. 1991. Sexual risk reduction behaviours among young heterosexual adults. Social Science and Medicine, 33, 25–36.

Cohen, J. 1995. Women: absent term in the AIDS research equation. Science, 269, 777–780.

Collazos V., C. 1994. Gender differentials and primary health care. In Wijeyaratne, P.; Hatcher Roberts, J.; Kitts, J.; Jones Arsenault, L., ed., Gender, health, and sustainable development: a Latin American perspective. Proceedings of a workshop held in Montevideo, Uruguay, 26–29 April 1994. International Development Research Centre, Ottawa, ON, Canada. pp. 185–193.

Committee of Asian Women. 1987. Health hazards of textile and garment industries. Asian Women Workers Newsletter (Hong Kong), 6(1), 1–2.

Commonwealth Secretariat. 1990. Engendering adjustment for the 1990s: report of the Commonwealth Expert Group on Women and Structural Adjustment. Commonwealth Secretariat, London, UK. 139 pp.

Conway, E.; Lambrou, Y. 1995. Gender and development: equity for all. IDRC Reports, 23(2), 4–7.

Conway, K. 1995. Soaps for social change. IDRC Reports, 23(2), 14.

Cook, R. 1994. Women's health and human rights. World Health Organization, Geneva, Switzerland. 62 pp.

Corlett, E.N.; Bishop, R.P. 1976. A technique for assessing postural discomfort. Ergonomics, 19, 175–192.

Cowley, G. 1992. A killer returns. Newsweek, 1992 (Nov.), pp. 34–39.
Crawford, M; Maracek, J. 1989. Psychology reconstructs the female. Psychology of Women Quarterly, 13, 147–165.

Danziger, R. 1994. The social impact of HIV/AIDS in developing countries. Social Science and Medicine, 39(7), 905–917.
Dawit, S. 1994. Ethics, gender, and health: a brief legal perspective. In Wijeyaratne, P.; Jones Arsenault, L.; Hatcher Roberts, J.; Kitts, J., ed., Gender, health, and sustainable development: proceedings of a workshop held in Nairobi, Kenya, 5–8 October 1993. International Development Research Centre, Ottawa, ON, Canada. pp. 173–178.
Debert-Ribeiro, M.B. 1993. Women and chronic diseases in Latin America. In Gómez Gómez, E., ed., Gender, women and health in the Americas. Pan American Health Organization, Washington, DC, USA. Scientific Publication 541, 82–89.
De Bruyn, M. 1992. Women and AIDS in developing countries. Social Science and Medicine, 34(3), 249–262.
———— 1993. Gender-related problems of self-protection against HIV infection. Vena Journal, 5(1), 6–11.
Dickson, K. 1995. A historical view of occupational health, gender, and sustainable development. In Hatcher Roberts, J.; Kitts, J.; Jones Arsenault, L., ed., Gender, health, and sustainable development: perspectives from Asia and the Caribbean. Proceedings of workshops held in Singapore, 23–26 January 1995, and in Bridgetown, Barbados, 6–9 December 1994. International Development Research Centre, Ottawa, ON, Canada. pp. 308–311.
DiClemente, R.J.; Durbin, M.; Siegel, D. 1992. Determinants of condom use among junior high school students in a minority inner-city school district. Pediatrics, 89, 197–920.
Diebel, L. 1995. Women harvest the grapes of NAFTA. Toronto Star, 27 May 1995, p. A18.
Dixon-Mueller, R.; Wasserheit, J. 1991. The culture of silence: reproductive tract infections among women in the Third World. International Women's Health Coalition, New York, NY, USA. 18 pp.
do Prado, E. 1994. Love does not protect against AIDS: reflections about the HIV/AIDS epidemic from a gender perspective. In Wijeyaratne, P.; Hatcher Roberts, J.; Kitts, J.; Jones Arsenault, L., ed., Gender, health, and sustainable development: a Latin American perspective. Proceedings of a workshop held in Montevideo, Uruguay, 26–29 April 1994. International Development Research Centre, Ottawa, ON, Canada. pp. 35–38.
Doty, P. 1987. Health status and health services use among older women: an international perspective. World Health Statistical Quarterly, 40, 279.
Duncan, M.E. 1992. Leprosy. In Wijeyaratne, P.; Rathgeber, E.M.; St.-Onge, E., ed., Women and tropical diseases. International Development Research Centre, Ottawa, ON, Canada. pp. 54–80.
Durana, C. 1994. Socioeconomic impact and gender differentials of cholera. In Wijeyaratne, P.; Hatcher Roberts, J.; Kitts, J.; Jones Arsenault, L., ed., Gender,

health, and sustainable development: a Latin American perspective. Proceedings from a workshop held in Montevideo, Uruguay, 26–29 April 1994. International Development Research Centre, Ottawa, ON, Canada. pp. 134–140.

Eagly, A.H.; Steffen, V.J. 1984. Gender stereotypes stem from the distribution of women and men into social roles. Journal of Personality and Social Psychology, 46, 735–754.

Eagly, A.H.; Wood, W. 1991. Explaining sex differences in social behaviour: a meta-analytic perspective. Personality and Social Psychology Bulletin, 17, 306–315.

Easterbrook, G. 1994. Forget PCB's, Radon, Alar: the world's greatest environmental dangers are dung smoke and dirty water. New York Times Magazine, 11 September 1994, Section 6, pp. 60–63.

Economist. 1994. The slaves from Myanmar. Economist, 5 February 1994, p. 32.

Eines, T. 1993. An analysis of the impact of Canadian health legislation on the well-being of women. In Gómez Gómez, E., ed., Gender, Women and health in the Americas. Pan American Health Organization, Washington, DC, USA. Scientific Publication 541, 225–236.

Eldemire, D. 1995. The elderly in Jamaica: a gender and development perspective. In Hatcher Roberts, J.; Kitts, J.; Jones Arsenault, L., ed., Gender, health, and sustainable development: perspectives from Asia and the Caribbean. Proceedings of workshops held in Singapore, 23–26 January 1995, and in Bridgetown, Barbados, 6–9 December 1994. International Development Research Centre, Ottawa, ON, Canada. pp. 291–296.

Elias, C.J. 1991. Sexually transmitted diseases and the reproductive health of women in developing countries. Population Council, New York, NY, USA. 54 pp.

Ellis, P. 1986. Methodologies for doing research on women and development. In Women in development: perspectives from the Nairobi conference. International Development Research Centre, Ottawa, ON, Canada. IDRC-MR137e, 136–143.

Engberg, L. 1993. Women and agricultural work. Occupational Medicine: State of the Art Reviews, 8(4), 869–882.

Espino, E. 1995. Women, children and malaria in the Philippines: would a community volunteer program work in their favour? In Hatcher Roberts, J.; Kitts, J.; Jones Arsenault, L., ed., Gender, health, and sustainable development: perspectives from Asia and the Caribbean. Proceedings of workshops held in Singapore, 23–26 January 1995, and in Bridgetown, Barbados, 6–9 December 1994. International Development Research Centre, Ottawa, ON, Canada. pp. 33–40.

Ettling, M. 1989. Evaluation of malaria clinics in Maesot, Thailand: use of serology to assess coverage. Transactions of the Royal Society of Tropical Medicine and Hygiene, 83, 320.

Ferguson, A. 1986. Women's health in a marginal area of Kenya. Social Science and Medicine, 23(1), 17–29.

Ferrando, J. 1992. Pensando en la educación popular (3rd ed.). Editorial Nordan-Communidad, Montevideo, Uruguay.

Ferrar, P. 1992. Food laced with cyanide. Partners in Reseach for Development (Australia), 5, 29–33.

Ford, N.; Koetsawang, S. 1991. The socio-cultural context of the transmission of HIV in Thailand. Social Science and Medicine, 33(4), 405–414.

Foreit, J.R.; Garate, M.R.; Brazzoduro, A.; Guillen, F.; Herrera, M. del Carmen; Suarez, F.C. 1992. A comparison of the performance of male and female CBD distributors in Peru. Studies in Family Planning, 23(1), 58–62.

Fraser, H.S. 1995. Impact of gender issues on chronic diseases. In Hatcher Roberts, J.; Kitts, J.; Jones Arsenault, L., ed., Gender, health, and sustainable development: perspectives from Asia and the Caribbean. Proceedings of workshops held in Singapore, 23–26 January 1995, and in Bridgetown, Barbados, 6–9 December 1994. International Development Research Centre, Ottawa, ON, Canada. pp. 350–352.

Garcia, R.; Antonio de Moya, E.; Fadul, R.; Freites, A.; Guerrero, S.; Castellanos, C.; 1994. Counsellors' and HIV-positive patients' perceptions of gender differences in HIV/AIDS education and counselling. In Wijeyaratne, P.; Hatcher Roberts, J.; Kitts, J.; Jones Arsenault, L., ed., Gender, health, and sustainable development: a Latin American perspective. Proceedings of a workshop held in Montevideo, Uruguay, 26–29 April 1994. International Development Research Centre, Ottawa, ON, Canada. pp. 39–50.

Gerelsuren, N.; Erdenechimeg, J. 1995. Mongolian women in health and development. In Hatcher Roberts, J.; Kitts, J.; Jones Arsenault, L., ed., Gender, health, and sustainable development: perspectives from Asia and the Caribbean. Proceedings of workshops held in Singapore, 23–26 January 1995, and in Bridgetown, Barbados, 6–9 December 1994. International Development Research Centre, Ottawa, ON, Canada. pp. 41–48.

Germain, A. 1991. Reproductive tract infections in women in the Third World: national and international policy implications. Report of a meeting at the Bellagio Study and Conference Center, 29 April–3 May 1991, Lake Como, Italy. Coalition, New York, NY, USA. 28 pp.

Gilligan, C. 1982. In a different voice: psychological theory and women's development. Harvard University Press, Cambridge, MA, USA. 184 pp.

Goldstein, D.M. 1994. AIDS and women in Brazil: the emerging problem. Social Science and Medicine, 39(7), 919–929.

Grandea, N. 1994. From blackboards to keyboards: the fragile link between women's education and employment. North–South Institute, Ottawa, ON, Canada. 63 pp.

Gray, L.A.; House, R.M. 1989. AIDS and adolescents. In Capuzzi D.; Gross D., ed., Working with at-risk youth: issues and interventions. American Association for Cooperation and Development, Alexandria, VA, USA.

Greaves, L.; Jordan, J.; McLellan, D. 1994. How tobacco touches women's lives. World Smoking and Health, 19(2), 2–3.

Greenhalgh, S. 1991. Women in the informal enterprise: empowerment or exploitation? Population Council, New York, NY, USA. Working Paper 33, 43 pp.

Guimarães, C.D. 1994. Male bisexuality, gender relations, and AIDS in Brazil. In Wijeyaratne, P.; Hatcher Roberts, J.; Kitts, J.; Jones Arsenault, L., ed., Gender, health, and sustainable development: a Latin American perspective. Proceedings of a workshop held in Montevideo, Uruguay, 26–29 April 1994. International Development Research Centre, Ottawa, ON, Canada. pp. 26–34.

Gupte, M. 1994. Initiatives by and for women through collective efforts. Paper presented at the workshop on the quality of health care for women in developing countries, 15–17 October 1994, Budapest, Hungary. World Health Organization, Geneva, Switzerland. 2 pp.

Gwede, C.; McDermott, R. 1992. AIDS in sub-Saharan Africa: implications for health education. AIDS Education and Prevention, 4(4), 350–361.

Haaland, A. 1994. Healthy women counselling guide: healthy communication with rural women. In Wijeyaratne, P.; Hatcher Roberts, J.; Kitts, J.; Jones Arsenault, L., ed., Gender, health, and sustainable development: a Latin American perspective. Proceedings of a workshop held in Montevideo, Uruguay, 26–29 April 1994. International Development Research Centre, Ottawa, ON, Canada. pp. 247–249.

Haile, F. 1985. Household energy in Addis Ababa: the supply and consumption of fuelwood. Addis Ababa Master Plan Project Office, Addis Ababa, Ethiopia.
———— 1994. Occupational participation of women and health. In Wijeyaratne, P.; Jones Arsenault, L.J.; Hatcher Roberts, J.; Kitts, J., ed., Gender, health, and sustainable development: proceedings of a workshop held in Nairobi, Kenya, 5–8 October 1993. International Development Research Centre, Ottawa, ON, Canada. pp. 129–135.

Hamblin, J.; Reid, E. 1991. Women, the HIV epidemic and human rights: a tragic imperative. Paper presented to the global meeting of experts on "AIDS: a question of rights and humanity," May 1991, The Hague, Netherlands. International Labour Organisation, Geneva, Switzerland.

Hammad, A.E.B. 1994. Introduction: opportunities and challenges for improving women's health status. In Wijeyaratne, P.; Hatcher Roberts, J.; Kitts, J.; Jones Arsenault, L., ed., Gender, health, and sustainable development: a Latin American perspective. Proceedings of a workshop held in Montevideo, Uruguay, 26–29 April 1994. International Development Research Centre, Ottawa, ON, Canada. pp. 1–5.

Hankins, C.; Handley, M. 1992. HIV disease and AIDS in women: current knowledge and a research agenda. Journal of Acquired Immune Deficiency Syndromes, 5(10), 957–971.

Hatcher Roberts, J.; Law, M. 1994. Poverty and powerlessness: an unhealthy combination for women in the developing world. Annals of the Royal College of Physicians and Surgeons of Canada (RCPSC), 27(6), 343–346.

Hazuda, H.P.; Haffner, S.; Stern, M.P. 1986. Employment status and women's protection against coronary heart disease. American Journal of Epidemiology, 123(4), 623–640.

Health and Welfare Canada. 1991. Health status of Canadian Indians and Inuit: 1990. Ministry of Supply and Services Canada, Ottawa, ON, Canada. 58 pp.

Heise, L. 1993. Violence against women. In Koblinsky, M.; Timyan, J.; Gay, J., ed., The health of women: a global perspective. Westview Press Inc., Boulder, CO, USA. pp. 171–195.

Heise, L.; Elias, C. 1995. Transforming AIDS prevention to meet women's needs: a focus on developing countries. Social Science and Medicine, 40(7), 931–943.

Hellandendu, J.M. 1992. Coping with physical disability: women's lives in rural Kilba Society. In Kissekka, M.N., ed., Women's Health Issues in Nigeria. Tamaza Publishing Company Ltd, Zaria, Nigeria. pp. 77–85.

Herrera, X.; Lobo-Guerrera, M. 1994. New models of participation in indigenous peoples' health. In Wijeyaratne, P.; Hatcher Roberts, J.; Kitts, J.; Jones Arsenault, L., ed., Gender, health, and sustainable development: a Latin American perspective. Proceedings of a workshop held in Montevideo, Uruguay, 26–29 April 1994. International Development Research Centre, Ottawa, ON, Canada. pp. 145–153.

Herrin, A.N. 1988. Perceptions of disease impacts: what can they tell us? In Herrin, A.N.; Rosenfield, P.L., ed., Economics, health and tropical diseases. School of Economics, University of the Philippines, Quezon City, Philippines. 470 pp.

Hollis, S. 1992. AIDS as a feminist issue. On the Level, 1(3), 15–18.

Holmboe-Ottesen, G.; Mascarenhas, O.; Wandel, M. 1989. Women's role in food chain activities and the implications for nutrition. United Nations Administration Committee on Coordination, Subcommittee on Nutrition, Geneva, Switzerland. State of the Art Series, Nutrition Policy Paper 4, 110 pp.

Hossain, H.R.J.; Sobhan, S. 1988. Industrialization and women workers in Bangladesh: from home-based work to the factories. In Heyzer, N., ed., Daughters in industry: work, skills and consciousness of women workers in Asia. Asian and Pacific Development Centre, Kuala Lumpur, Malaysia. 395 pp.

Htoon, M.T.; Bertolli, J.; Kosasih, L.D. 1993. Leprosy. In Jamieson, D.T.; Mosley, W.H.; Measham, A.R.; Bobadilla, J.L., ed., Disease control priorities in developing countries. Oxford Medical Publications, London, UK. pp. 261–280.

Huang, Y.; Manderson, L. 1992. Schistosomiasis and the social patterning of infection. Acta Tropica, 51, 175–194.

Humphrey, J. 1987. Gender and work in the Third World: sexual divisions in Brazilian society. Tavistock Publications, London, UK. 229 pp.

ICRW (International Center for Research on Women). 1989. Strengthening women: health research priorities for women in developing countries. ICRW, Washington, DC, USA. 70 pp.

IHT (International Herald Tribune). 1993. Thai fire shows seamy side of growth. International Herald Tribune, 13 May 1993, p. 15.

Illo, J.F.I. 1991. Looking at gender and development: an analytical framework. Partnerships: Bulletin of the Philippine Development Assistance Programme, 5(2), 1–8.

ILO (International Labour Organisation). 1985. World Labour Report 1985, ILO, Geneva, Switzerland. 245 pp.

———— 1989. Special protective measures for women and equality of opportunity and treatment. Documents considered at the meeting of experts on special protective measures for women and equality of opportunity and treatment. ILO, Geneva, Switzerland. MEPMW/1989/7, 87 pp.

———— 1992a. World labour report 1992. ILO, Geneva, Switzerland. 105 pp.

———— 1992b. Homeworkers of Southeast Asia: the struggle for social protection in Thailand. ILO Regional Office for Asia and the Pacific, Bangkok, Thailand. 225 pp.

———— 1993. Unequal race to the top. World of Work: the Magazine of the ILO, 2, 6–7.

———— 1994. World labour report 1994. ILO, Geneva, Switzerland. 113 pp.

Iqbal, T. 1995. Education, gender, and relationships between female clients and health providers. In Hatcher Roberts, J.; Vlassoff, C., ed., The female client and the health-care provider. International Development Research Centre, Ottawa, ON, Canada. p. 157.

Islam, S. 1989. The socio-cultural context of childbirth in rural Bangladesh. In Krishnaraj, M.; Chanana, K., ed., Gender and the household domain: social and cultural dimensions. Sage Publications, New Delhi, India.

Jacobson, J.L. 1992a. The other epidemic. World Watch, 5(3), 10–17.

———— 1992b. Out of the woods. World Watch, 5(6), 26–31.

———— 1993. Women's health: the price of poverty. In Koblinsky, M.; Timyan, J.; Gay, J., ed., The health of women: a global perspective. Westview Press Inc., Boulder, CO, USA. pp. 3–31.

Jacquette, J. 1986. Female political participation in Latin America: raising feminist issues. In Iglitzin, L.B.; Ross, R., ed., Women in the world 1975–1985: the women's decade. ABC-Cio, Santa Barbara, CA, USA. pp. 243–269.

Janzen, J.M. 1978. The quest for therapy — medical pluralism in Lower Zaire: comparative studies of health systems and medical care. University of California Press, Berkeley, CA, USA. 266 pp.

Jay, S.; Bridges, C.E.; Gottlieb, A.A.; DuRant, R.H. 1988. Factors related to behavior change in response to AIDS. Family Relations, 41, 97–103.

Jeffery, P.; Jeffery, R.; Lyon, A. 1988. Labour pains and labour power: women and childbearing in India. Zed Books Ltd, London, UK. 292 pp.

Johnson Controls. 1991. International Union, United Automobile, Aerospace and Agricultural Implement Workers of America, UAW vs. Johnson Controls. Supreme Court Reporter (US), 11, 1196–1216.

Johnson, L. 1982. The seam allowance: industrial home sewing in Canada. Women's Press, Toronto, ON, Canada. 135 pp.

Jones, L.; Catalan, J. 1989. Women and HIV disease. British Journal of Hospital Medicine, 41, 526–538.

Joyce, K. 1988. Internal and external barriers to obtaining prenatal care. In Brown S.,
ed., Prenatal care: reaching mothers, reaching infants. National Academy
Press, Washington, DC, USA. 254 pp.

Kaendi, J.M. 1994. Gender issues in the prevention and control of visceral leischma-
niasis. In Wijeyaratne, P.; Jones Arsenault, L.; Hatcher Roberts, J.; Kitts, J.,
ed., Gender, health, and sustainable development: proceedings of a workshop
held in Nairobi, Kenya, 5–8 October 1993. International Development
Research Centre, Ottawa, ON, Canada. pp. 110–116.

Kambon, A. 1995. Multiculturalism: women, HIV/AIDS and development. In
Hatcher Roberts, J.; Kitts, J.; Jones Arsenault, L., ed., Gender, health, and sus-
tainable development: perspectives from Asia and the Caribbean. Proceedings
of workshops held in Singapore, 23–26 January 1995, and in Bridgetown,
Barbados, 6–9 December 1994. International Development Research Centre,
Ottawa, ON, Canada. pp. 315–325.

Kaseje, D.C.O.; Sempebwa, E.K.; Spencer, H.C. 1987. Malaria chemoprophylaxis to
pregnant women provided by community health workers in Saradidi, Kenya. I.
Reasons for non-acceptance. Annals of Tropical Medicine and Parasitology,
81(Suppl. 1), 1.

Keeling, R.P. 1993. Commentary: education and counselling about HIV in the second decade. Journal of Counselling and Development, 71, 306–309.

Kerawalla, G.J. 1994. Educational status of girls: an inquiry into gender and
urban/rural disparities. Paper presented at the national seminar on update on
status of adolescent girls: initiatives and progress in India, September 1994.
SNDT Women's University, Bombay, India.

Kettel, B. 1996. Women, health and the environment. Social Science and Medicine
(Special issue on women and health policy in development). In press.

Khan, Z.H.; Midhet, F. 1991. Women's and infants' mortality and morbidity during
and after harvest season in rural Pakistan. Paper presented at the 18th annual
National Council for International Health Conference, June 1991, Arlington,
VA, USA.

Klugman, B. 1994. Feminist methodology in relation to the women's health project.
In Wijeyaratne, P.; Jones Arsenault, L.; Hatcher Roberts, J.; Kitts, J., ed.,
Gender, health, and sustainable development: proceedings of a workshop held
in Nairobi, Kenya, 5–8 October 1993. International Development Research
Centre, Ottawa, ON, Canada. pp. 187–204.

Koblinsky, M.; Campbell, O.M.R.; Harlow, S.D. 1993. Mother and more: a broader
perspective on women's health. In Koblinsky, M.; Timyan, J.; Gay, J., ed., The
health of women: a global perspective. Westview Press Inc., Boulder, CO,
USA. pp. 33–62.

Koblinsky, M.; Timyan, J.; Gay, J., ed., 1993. The health of women: a global perspective. Westview Press Inc., Boulder, CO, USA.

Kumar, S.K.; Hotchkiss, D. 1988. Consequences of deforestation for women's time
allocation, agricultural production, and nutrition in hill areas of Nepal.
International Food Policy Research Institute, Washington, DC, USA. 72 pp.

Kurppa, K.; Waris, P.; Rokkanen, P. 1979. Peritendinitis and tenosynovitis: a review. Scandinavian Journal of Work, Environment and Health, 5(3), 19–24.

Kuyyakonond, T. 1995. The role of rural women in AIDS prevention and control. In Hatcher Roberts, J.; Kitts, J.; Jones Arsenault, L. Gender, health, and sustainable development: perspectives from Asia and the Caribbean. Proceedings of workshops held in Singapore, 23–26 January 1995, and in Bridgetown, Barbados, 6–9 December 1994. International Development Research Centre, Ottawa, ON, Canada. pp. 58–68.

Kwawu, J. 1994. Gender and household health seeking behaviours. In Wijeyaratne, P.; Jones Arsenault, L.; Hatcher Roberts, J.; Kitts, J., ed., Gender, health, and sustainable development: proceedings of a workshop held in Nairobi, Kenya, 5–8 October 1993. International Development Research Centre, Ottawa, ON, Canada. pp. 225–229.

Labour Resource Centre. 1995. Engendering occupational health and safety. In Hatcher Roberts, J.; Kitts, J.; Jones Arsenault, L. Gender, health, and sustainable development: perspectives from Asia and the Caribbean. Proceedings of workshops held in Singapore, 23–26 January 1995, and in Bridgetown, Barbados, 6–9 December 1994. International Development Research Centre, Ottawa, ON, Canada. pp. 69–78.

LaDou, J. 1993. Women workers: international issues. Occupational Medicine: State of the Art Reviews, 8(4), 673–683.

Lane, S.D.; Meleis, A.I. 1991. Roles, work, health perceptions and health resources of women: a study in an Egyptian delta hamlet. Social Science and Medicine, 33(10), 1197–1208.

Lange, I.; Aguilo, A.; Barros, C. 1994. Health promoters: invisible providers of care. In Wijeyaratne, P.; Hatcher Roberts, J.; Kitts, J.; Jones Arsenault, L., ed., Gender, health, and sustainable development: a Latin American perspective. Proceedings of a workshop held in Montevideo, Uruguay, 26–29 April 1994. International Development Research Centre, Ottawa, ON, Canada. pp. 194–198.

Larson, A. 1990. The social epidemiology of Africa's AIDS epidemic. African Affairs, 89(354), 5–26.

Law, M. 1994. Introduction. In Wijeyaratne, P.; Jones Arsenault, L.; Hatcher Roberts, J.; Kitts, J., ed., Gender, health, and sustainable development: proceedings of a workshop held in Nairobi, Kenya, 5–8 October 1993. International Development Research Centre, Ottawa, ON, Canada. pp. 1–2.

Lee, C.; Duxbury, L.; Higgins, C. 1994. Employed mothers: balancing work and family life. Supply and Services Canada, Ottawa, ON, Canada. 42 pp.

Lee, S.H. 1984. Occupational and health hazards with special reference to female workers. Paper presented at a seminar on women and employment, 16–17 April 1984, Kuala Lumpur, Malaysia. Asian and Pacific Development Centre, Kuala Lumpur, Malayia. 15 pp.

Lema, V.M.; Kabeberi-Macharia, J. 1992. A review of abortion in Kenya. English Press Ltd, Nairobi, Kenya.

Leslie, J. 1992. Women's lives and women's health: using social science research to promote better health for women. International Center for Research on Women, Washington, DC, USA. 40 pp.

Leslie J.; Lucette M.; Buvinic M. 1988. Weathering economic crises: the crucial role of women in health. In Bell, D.; Reich, M., ed., Health, nutrition and the economic crises: approaches to policy in the Third World. Auburn House, Dover, MA, USA. pp. 307–348.

Lim, L.L. 1988. Economic dynamist and structural transformation in the Asian Pacific rim countries: contributions of the second sex. Nihon University Population Research Institute, Tokyo, Japan. NUPRI Research Paper Series 45, 37 pp.

Lopez-Gonzaga, V. 1995. The story of Myrna Colantro. In Hatcher Roberts, J.; Kitts, J.; Jones Arsenault, L., ed., Gender, health and sustainable development: perspectives from Asia and the Caribbean. Proceedings of workshops held in Singapore, 23–26 January 1995, and in Bridgetown, Barbados, 6–9 December 1994. International Development Research Centre, Ottawa, ON, Canada. pp. 13–14.

Lorber, J. 1984. Women physicians: careers, status, and power. Tavistock Publications, New York, NY, USA. 149 pp.

Lowe, G. 1989. Le travail de femmes et le stress. Conseil consultatif Canadian sur la situation de la femme, Ottawa, ON, Canada. 89 pp.

Lule, G.; Ssembatya, M. 1995. Intention to delivery and delivery outcome. In Hatcher Roberts, J.; Vlassoff, C. ed., The female client and the health-care provider. International Development Research Centre, Ottawa, ON, Canada. pp. 79–90.

Luppi, I. 1994. Women's perspectives on health/illness processes and the response of health care services. Paper presented at the workshop on the quality of health care for women in developing countries, 15–17 October 1994, Budapest, Hungary. World Health Organization, Geneva, Switzerland. 14 pp.

Lwihula, G.K. 1994. Gender and acceptance of medical innovations and technologies related to STDs and AIDS in Africa. In Wijeyaratne, P.; Jones Arsenault, L.; Hatcher Roberts, J.; Kitts, J., ed., Gender, health, and sustainable development: proceedings of a workshop held in Nairobi, Kenya, 5–8 October 1993. International Development Research Centre, Ottawa, ON, Canada. pp. 59–65.

MacCormack, C. 1992. Planning and evaluating women's participation in primary health care. Social Science and Medicine, 35(6), 831–837.

Machado, M.H. 1993. Women and the health sector's labor market in the Americas: female hegemony? In Gómez Gómez, E., ed., Gender, women and health in the Americas. Pan American Health Organization, Washington, DC, USA. Scientific Publication 541, 255–262.

MacMillan, N. 1995. Ecuador: health and the working woman. IDRC Reports, 23(2), 10–11.

Manderson, L. 1994. Expanding quality of care beyond reproductive health. Paper presented at the workshop on the quality of health care for women in developing countries, 15–17 October 1994, Budapest, Hungary. World Health Organization, Geneva, Switzerland. 6 pp.

Manderson, L.; Jenkins, J.; Tanner, M. 1993. Women and tropical diseases: an introduction. Social Science and Medicine, 37(4), 441–443.

Mantell, J.; Schinke, S.; Akabas, S. 1988. Women and AIDS prevention. Journal of Primary Prevention, 9(1/2), 18–40.

March, K.S.; Taqqu, R. 1982. Women's informal associations and the organizational capacity for development. Center for International Studies, Cornell University, Ithaca, NY, USA. Monograph Series 5.

Mata, L. 1982. Sociocultural factors in the control and prevention of parasitic diseases. Review of Infectious Diseases, 4(4), 871–879.

Mawajdeh, S.; Al-Qutob, R.; Raad, F.B. 1995. The assessment of quality of care in prenatal services in Irbid, North Jordan: women's perspectives. In Hatcher Roberts, J.; Vlassoff, C. ed., The female client and the health-care provider. International Development Research Centre, Ottawa, ON, Canada. pp. 1–18.

Mbacke, C.; van de Walle, E. 1987. Socio-economic factors and access to health services as determinants of child mortality: IUSSP seminar on mortality and society in sub-Saharan Africa, Yaoundé, Cameroon. International Union for the Scientific Study of Population, Liège, Belgium.

McCauley, A.P.; West, S.; Lynch, M. 1992. Household decisions among the Gogo people of Tanzania: determining the roles of men, women and the community in implementing a trachoma prevention program. Social Science and Medicine, 34(7), 817–824.

McCord, C.; Freeman, H.P. 1990. Excess mortality in Harlem. New England Journal of Medicine, 322(3), 173–177.

McDaniel, S.A. 1987. Women, work and health: some challenges to health promotion. Canadian Journal of Public Health, 78, S9–S13.

McGuire, J.S.; Popkin, B.M. 1989. Beating the zero-sum game: women and nutrition in the Third World — Part I. Food and Nutrition Bulletin, 11, 38–63.

Mechanic, D. 1976. Sex, illness, illness behaviour, and the use of health services. Social Science and Medicine, 12B, 207–214.

Medel, J.; Riquelme, V. 1992. Mujer, trabajo y salud: las trabajadoras asalariadas de la fruticultura. Centro de Estudios de la Mujer, Santiago, Chile.

Melnick, S.L.; Sherer, R.; Louis, T.A.; Hillman, D. 1994. Survival and disease progression according to gender of patients with HIV infection: the Terry Beirn Community Programs for Clinical Research on AIDS. Journal of the American Medical Association, 272(24), 1915–1921.

Mencher, J.P. 1988. Women's work and poverty: women's contribution to household maintenance in South India. In Dwyer, D.; Bruce, J., ed., A home divided: women and income in the Third World. Stanford University Press, Stanford, CA, USA. pp. 99–119.

Meng, K.-H.; Lee, B.K.; Park, C.Y.; Lee, W.C.; Cho, H.S. 1987. Occupational health risks of female workers of manufacturing industries in Korea. Catholic Industrial Medical Center, Catholic University Medical College, Seoul, Korea.

Messing, K. 1991. Occupational safety and health concerns of Canadian women: a background paper. Supply and Services Canada, Ottawa, ON, Canada. 96 pp.

———— 1994. Women's occupational health and androcentric science. Canadian Women's Studies, 14(3), 11–16.

Mhloyi, G.D.; Mhloyi, M.M. 1994. Socio-cultural determinants of HIV infection in Zimbabwe. In Wijeyaratne, P.; Jones Arsenault, L.; Hatcher Roberts, J.; Kitts, J., ed., Gender, health, and sustainable development: proceedings of a workshop held in Nairobi, Kenya, 5–8 October 1993. International Development Research Centre, Ottawa, ON, Canada. pp. 9–20.

Michelson, E.H. 1992. Adam's rib awry: women and schistosomiasis. In Wijeyaratne, P.; Rathgeber, E.M.; St.-Onge, E., ed., Women and tropical diseases. International Development Research Centre, Ottawa, ON, Canada. pp. 24–40.

Milio, N. 1986. Promoting health through public policy. Canadian Public Health Association, Ottawa, ON, Canada. 359 pp.

Misch, A. 1992. Lost in the shadow economy. World Watch, 5(2), 18–25.

Mitter, S. 1986. Common fate, common bond: women in the global economy. Pluto Press, London, UK. 119 pp.

———— 1994. A comparative survey. In Martens, M.H.; Mitter, S., ed., Women in trade unions: organizing the unorganized. International Labour Organisation, Geneva, Switzerland. pp. 3–14.

Momsen, J.H. 1991. Women and development in the Third World. Routledge and Kegan Paul, London, UK. 115 pp.

Moore, D.M. 1981. Assertiveness training: a review. In Cox, S., ed., Female psychology: the emerging self. St Martin's Press, New York, NY, USA. 494 pp.

Morris, M.; Pramualratana, A.; Podhisita, C.; Wawer, M. 1994. The relational determinants of condom use in Thailand. Center for Population and Family Health, Columbia University, New York, NY, USA. Report 10.

Mpanju, W.F. 1992. Women in health: maternal nutrition and reproductive health. Paper presented at the first international conference of social science and medicine, 10–13 August 1992. Africa Network (SOMA-NET), Nairobi, Kenya.

Mull, J.D.; Wood, C.S.; Gans, L.P.; Mull, D.S. 1989. Culture and "compliance" among leprosy patients in Pakistan. Social Science and Medicine, 29(7), 799–811.

Muntemba, S. 1989. Women and environment in Africa: towards a conceptualization. In Rathgeber, E.M., ed., Women's role in natural resource management in Africa. International Development Research Centre, Ottawa, ON, Canada. IDRC-MR238e, 1–5.

Mutinga, J.M. 1984. Epidemiological investigations of visceral leishmaniasis in West Pokot District, Kenya. Insect Science and Application, 5(6).

Mwenesi, H.A. 1994. Women and decision-making for their children's health care. In Wijeyaratne, P.; Jones Arsenault, L.; Hatcher Roberts, J.; Kitts, J., ed., Gender, health, and sustainable development: proceedings of a workshop held in Nairobi, Kenya, 5–8 October 1993. International Development Research Centre, Ottawa, ON, Canada. pp. 117–126.

Nájera, J.A.; Liese, B.H.; Hammer, J. 1993. Malaria. In Jamieson, D.T.; Mosley, W.H.; Measham, A.R.; Bobadilla, J.L., ed., Disease control priorities in developing countries. Oxford Medical Publications, London, UK. pp. 281–302.

Nandy, A.; Addy, M.; Chowdhury, A.; Ghosh, A. 1988. Current state of visceral leishmaniasis in India with special reference to West Bengal. In Walton, B.C.; Wijeyaratne, P.; Modabber, F., ed., Research on control strategies for the leishmaniasis: proceedings of an international workshop held in Ottawa, Canada, 1–4 June 1987. International Development Research Centre, Ottawa, ON, Canada. IDRC-MR184e, 8–15.

Nayak-Mukherjee, V. 1991. Women in the economy: a selected annotated bibliography of Asia and Pacific. Asian and Pacific Development Centre, Kuala Lumpur, Malaysia. 156 pp.

NCSEW (National Commission on Self-Employed Women). 1988. Occupational health issues of women in the unorganized sector: report of the Task Force of Health. NCSEW, Bombay, India.

Ndejembi, E. 1993. Ignorance and AIDS myths "rife." WorldAIDS, 30, 4.

Ndhlovu, L. 1994. Clients' and providers' definitions and perspectives of quality of family planning services. Paper presented at the workshop on the quality of health care for women in developing countries, 15–17 October 1994, Budapest, Hungary. World Health Organization, Geneva, Switzerland. 29 pp.

New York Times. 1995. AIDS cases rising sharply among women. New York Times, 10 February 1995, p. 11.

Nga, N.N. 1995. Selected aspects of women's working conditions in Vietnam. In Hatcher Roberts, J.; Kitts, J.; Jones Arsenault, L., ed., Gender, health, and sustainable development: perspectives from Asia and the Caribbean. Proceedings of workshops held in Singapore, 23–26 January 1996, and in Bridgetown, Barbados, 6–9 December 1994. International Development Research Centre, Ottawa, ON, Canada. pp. 90–95.

Ngugi, E. 1991. Education and counseling interventions. Paper presented at the 18th annual National Council for International Health Conference, Arlington, VA, USA.

Ngwenya, S. 1994. Implementing issues in gender and health: emphasizing STDs in rural South Africa. In Wijeyaratne, P.; Jones Arsenault, L.; Hatcher Roberts, J.; Kitts, J., ed., Gender, health, and sustainable development: proceedings of a workshop held in Nairobi, Kenya, 5–8 October 1993. International Development Research Centre, Ottawa, ON, Canada. pp. 66–74.

Niraula, B.B. 1994. Use of health services in hill villages in Central Nepal. Health Transitions Review, 4, 151–166.

Nowak, R. 1995. Rockefeller's big prize for STD test. Science, 269, 782.

Nuss, S. 1989. Women in the world of work: statistical analysis and projections to the year 2000. International Labour Organisation, Geneva, Switzerland. 132 pp.

O'Connor, P.; Leshabari, M.T.; Lwihula, G.K. 1992. Ethnographic study of the truck stops environment in Tanzania. Family Health International, Durham, NC, USA.

Oh, K. 1995. Abortion experiences of Korean women and the implications for public policy. In Hatcher Roberts, J.; Kitts, J.; Jones Arsenault, L., ed., Gender, health, and sustainable development: perspectives from Asia and the Caribbean. Proceedings of workshops held in Singapore, 23–26 January 1995, and in Bridgetown, Barbados, 6–9 December 1994. International Development Research Centre, Ottawa, ON, Canada. pp. 97–105.

Okojie, C.E.E. 1994. Gender inequities of health in the Third World. Social Science and Medicine, 39(9), 1237–1247.

Omer Haski, K.; Silver, J. 1994. No words can express: two voices on female genital mutilation. Canadian Woman Studies, 14(3), 62–65.

Ortiz, P.J. July 1994. Keeping it safe. WorldAIDS, 34, 2.

Osteria, T.S. 1995. Gender, reproductive health, and sustainable development: the Philippine context. In Hatcher Roberts, J.; Kitts, J.; Jones Arsenault, L., ed., Gender, health, and sustainable development: perspectives from Asia and the Caribbean. Proceedings of workshops held in Singapore, 23–26 January 1995, and in Bridgetown, Barbados, 6–9 December 1994. International Development Research Centre, Ottawa, ON, Canada. pp. 106–121.

Pagé, L. 1995. Women: the handymen of South Africa. IDRC Reports, 23(2), 8–9.

PAHO; WHO (Pan American Health Organization; World Health Organization). 1992. The health of women in the English-speaking Caribbean. PAHO, Washington, DC, USA. 31 pp.

Panos Institute. 1990. Triple jeopardy: women and AIDS. Panos Institute, London, UK. 104 pp.

———— 1992. Breaking the chain: STDs and HIV. WorldAIDS, 22, 5–8.

———— 1994a. On the brink. WorldAIDS, 31, 6–9.

———— 1994b. Dangerous practices. WorldAIDS, 33, 5–9.

Paolisso, M. 1995. New directions for the study of women and environmental degradation. International Center for Research on Women, Washington, DC, USA. 15 pp.

Paolisso, M.; Blumberg, R.L. 1989. Women in development: recommendations for future activities. International Center for Research on Women, Washington, DC, USA.

Paolisso, M.; Leslie, J. 1995. Meeting the changing health needs of women in developing countries. Social Science and Medicine, 40(1), 55–65.

Parker, M. 1992. Does schistosomiasis infection impair the health of women? In Wijeyaratne, P.; Rathgeber, E.M.; St.-Onge, E., ed., Women and tropical diseases. International Development Research Centre, Ottawa, ON, Canada. pp. 81–99.

Patrick, W.K. 1991. The impact of manufacturing industries on the status of health of women. Paper presented at the 18th annual National Council for International Health Conference, Arlington, VA, USA.

Patterson, A.W. 1995. Gender and nutrition. In Hatcher Roberts, J.; Kitts, J.; Jones Arsenault, L., ed., Gender, health, and sustainable development: perspectives from Asia and the Caribbean. Proceedings of workshops held in Singapore, 23–26 January 1995, and in Bridgetown, Barbados, 6–9 December 1994.

International Development Research Centre, Ottawa, ON, Canada. pp. 285–290.

Pauw, I. 1993. Commercial sex workers: towards an understanding. AIDS Bulletin, 2(1), 12–13.

Peacocke, N. 1995. WAND, promoting behaviour change, and gender. In Hatcher Roberts, J.; Kitts, J.; Jones Arsenault, L., ed., Gender, health, and sustainable development: perspectives from Asia and the Caribbean. Proceedings of workshops held in Singapore, 23–26 January 1995, and in Bridgetown, Barbados, 6–9 December 1994. International Development Research Centre, Ottawa, ON, Canada. pp. 277–279.

Pearlberg, G. 1991. Women, AIDS and communities: a guide for action. Women's Action Alliance Inc., New York, NY, USA. 129 pp.

Perlez, J. 1990. For the oppressed sex: brave words to live by. New York Times, 6 June 1990, p. A4.

Pesce, L. 1994. AIDS research from a gender perspective. In Wijeyaratne, P.; Hatcher Roberts, J.; Kitts, J.; Jones Arsenault, L., ed., Gender, health, and sustainable development: a Latin American perspective. Proceedings of a workshop held in Montevideo, Uruguay, 26–29 April 1994. International Development Research Centre, Ottawa, ON, Canada. pp. 19–25.

Pinel, A. 1994. Besides carnival and soccer: reflections about AIDS in Brazil. In Wijeyaratne, P.; Hatcher Roberts, J.; Kitts, J.; Jones Arsenault, L., ed., Gender, health, and sustainable development: a Latin American perspective. Proceedings of a workshop held in Montevideo, Uruguay, 26–29 April 1994. International Development Research Centre, Ottawa, ON, Canada. pp. 62–71.

Pino, P.; Florenzano, R.; Nudman, A. 1994. Sexual initiation of school-age adolescents in Santiago, Chile: the implications of gender, religion, and family structure. In Wijeyaratne, P.; Hatcher Roberts, J.; Kitts, J.; Jones Arsenault, L., ed., Gender, health, and sustainable development: a Latin American perspective. Proceedings of a workshop held in Montevideo, Uruguay, 26–29 April 1994. International Development Research Centre, Ottawa, ON, Canada. pp. 51–61.

Planning Institute of Jamaica. 1989. Economic and social survey Jamaica. Planning Institute of Jamaica, Kingston, Jamaica.

Pleck, J. 1985. Working wives/working husbands. Sage, Newbury Park, CA, USA. 167 pp.

Population Reports. 1990. Condoms — now more than ever. Population Information Program, Johns Hopkins School of Hygiene and Public Health, Baltimore, MD, USA. Barrier Methods, Series H, 8, 35 pp.

Pradubmook P. 1994. The social dimensions of condom use among female commercial sex workers in Thailand: a qualitative analysis. Paper presented at the 2nd Asia–Pacific Social Science and Medicine Conference, May 1994, Manilla, Philippines.

Pramualratana, A. 1995. Husband and wife dynamics and barriers to condom use: issues to consider. In Hatcher Roberts, J.; Kitts, J.; Jones Arsenault, L., ed., Gender, health, and sustainable development: perspectives from Asia and the

Caribbean. Proceedings of workshops held in Singapore, 23–26 January 1995, and in Bridgetown, Barbados, 6–9 December 1994. International Development Research Centre, Ottawa, ON, Canada. pp. 126–134.

Priest, L. 1994. Most medical research ignores women patients. Toronto Star, 6 November 1994, p. A1.

Prompunthum, V.; Kerdpol, C. 1985. Working conditions of women piece-rate workers in Thailand. United Nations Economic and Social Commission for Asia and the Pacific, Bangkok, Thailand.

Punnett, L. 1985. Soft tissue disorders in the upper limbs of female garment workers. Scandinavian Journal of Work, Environment and Health, 11, 417–425.

Puta, A.K. 1994. Occupational health, safety and gender. In Wijeyaratne, P.; Jones Arsenault, L.; Hatcher Roberts, J.; Kitts, J., ed., Gender, health, and sustainable development: proceedings of a workshop held in Nairobi, Kenya, 5–8 October 1993. International Development Research Centre, Ottawa, ON, Canada. pp. 163–170.

Ramazanoglu, C. 1989. Feminism and the contradictions of oppression. Routledge and Kegan Paul, London, UK. 218 pp.

Ramphele, M.; Boonzaier, E. 1988. The position of African women: race and gender in South Africa. In Boonzaier E.; Sharp, J., ed., South African keywords: the uses and abuses of political concepts. David Philip, Cape Town, South Africa. pp. 153–166.

Rana, S. 1991. The sex worker and the market. HIMAL, 4(4), 17–20.

Rathgeber, E.M. 1990a. Integrating gender into development: research and action agendas for the 1990s. International Development Research Centre, Ottawa, ON, Canada. Mimeo.

———— 1990b. WID, WAD, GAD: trends in research and practice. Journal of Developing Areas, 24, 489–502.

———— 1994a. Special issues to consider when doing research on women. In Wijeyaratne, P.; Jones Arsenault, L.; Hatcher Roberts, J.; Kitts, J., ed., Gender, health, and sustainable development: proceedings of a workshop held in Nairobi, Kenya, 5–8 October 1993. International Development Research Centre, Ottawa, ON, Canada. pp. 271–274.

———— 1994b. Operationalizing gender and development. International Development Research Centre, Ottawa, ON, Canada. 30 pp. Mimeo.

Rathgeber, E.M.; Vlassoff, C. 1993. Gender and tropical diseases: a new research focus. Social Science and Medicine, 37(4), 513–520.

RCNRT (Royal Commission on New Reproductive Technologies). 1993. Proceed with care: final report of the Royal Commission on New Reproductive Technologies. Supply and Services Canada, Ottawa, ON, Canada. 1275 pp.

Ren, N.; Khieu, S.V.; Chhoy, K.S. 1995. Women's health in Cambodia. In Hatcher Roberts, J.; Kitts, J.; Jones Arsenault, L., ed., Gender, health, and sustainable development: perspectives from Asia and the Caribbean. Proceedings of workshops held in Singapore, 23–26 January 1995, and in Bridgetown, Barbados, 6–9 December 1994. International Development Research Centre, Ottawa, ON, Canada. pp. 79–84.

Repetti, R.L.; Mathews, K.A.; Waldron, I. 1989. Employment and women's health: effects of paid employment on women's mental and physical health. American Psychologist, 44(11), 1394–1401.

Reubin, R. 1992. Women and malaria. In Wijeyaratne, P.; Rathgeber, E.M.; St.-Onge, E., ed., Women and tropical diseases. International Development Research Centre, Ottawa, ON, Canada. pp. 41–53.

Richters, A. 1994. Building a new paradigm: gender, health and development. Women's Health Journal (ISIS International), 2–3, 40–46.

Rodin, J.; Ickovics, J. 1990. Women's health. Review and research agenda as we approach the 21st century. American Psychologist, 45(9), 1018–1034.

Rodney, P. 1995. The state, gender, and health care services: Barbados and Grenada 1979–1983. In Hatcher Roberts, J.; Kitts, J.; Jones Arsenault, L., ed., Gender, health, and sustainable development: perspectives from Asia and the Caribbean. Proceedings of workshops held in Singapore, 23–26 January 1995, and in Bridgetown, Barbados, 6–9 December 1994. International Development Research Centre, Ottawa, ON, Canada. pp. 262–276.

Rogler, L.H. 1989. The meaning of culturally sensitive research in mental health. American Journal of Psychiatry, 146, 296–303.

Rojas, J.G. 1992. Family feeding and commercial production: a theoretical reflection for a documentary framework on health. Paper presented at the 2nd Seminar on the Evaluation of Projects of the Etnollano Foundation. Etnollano Foundation, Villa de Leyva, Colombia.

Rosser, S. 1991. AIDS and women. AIDS Education and Prevention, 3(3), 230–240.

Rowbotham, S. 1993. Homeworkers worldwide. Merlin Press, London, UK. 92 pp.

Rozario, S. 1995. Dai and midwives: the renegotiation of the status of birth attendants in contemporary Bangladesh. In Hatcher Roberts, J.; Vlassoff, C., ed., The female client and the health-care provider. International Development Research Centre, Ottawa, ON, Canada. pp. 92–112.

Sacco, W.P.; Rickman, R.L.; Thompson, K.; Levine, B.; Reed, D.L. 1993. Gender differences in AIDS-relevant condom attitudes and condom use. AIDS Education and Prevention, 5(4), 311–326.

Sachs, A. 1994. Men, sex, and parenthood in an overpopulating world. World Watch, 7(2), 12–19.

Salinas, J. 1988. Experiencias de participación communitaria en salud y nutrición: notas para un analisis. Review of Child Nutrition, 16(3), 279–285.

Sarti, E.J. 1994. Considerations for the control and prevention of neurocysticercosis. In Wijeyaratne, P.; Hatcher Roberts, J.; Kitts, J.; Jones Arsenault, L., ed., Gender, health, and sustainable development: a Latin American perspective. Proceedings of a workshop held in Montevideo, Uruguay, 26–29 April 1994. International Development Research Centre, Ottawa, ON, Canada. pp. 107–114.

Schoepf, B. 1988. Women, AIDS, and economic crisis in Central Africa. Canadian Journal of African Studies, 22(3), 625–644.

———— 1993. AIDS action-research with women in Kinshasa, Zaire. Social Science and Medicine, 37(11), 1401–1413.

Sekimpi, D.K. 1988. Acquired immunodeficiency syndrome (AIDS) and occupational health in Uganda. In Fleming, A., ed., The global impact of AIDS. Alan R. Liss Inc., New York, NY, USA.

Seraprespamni, T. 1991. Risk factors for HIV among prostitutes in Chiangmai, Thailand. AIDS, 5, 579–582.

Sermsri, S. 1995. Does education empower women for health and sustainable development? In Hatcher Roberts, J.; Kitts, J.; Jones Arsenault, L., ed., Gender, health, and sustainable development: perspectives from Asia and the Caribbean. Proceedings of workshops held in Singapore, 23–26 January 1995, and in Bridgetown, Barbados, 6–9 December 1994. International Development Research Centre, Ottawa, ON, Canada. pp. 135–138.

Serrill, M.S. 1995. Domestic violence: a death sentence for a young Filipino maid highlights the problems of abuse of Asian servants. Time International, 23 October 1995, pp. 57–59.

Shenon, P. 1993. Thai fire inquiry sees arson or negligence. International Herald Tribune, 14 May 1993, p. 2.

Silva, K.T. 1988. Malaria control through community action at the grass-roots: experience of the Sarvodaya malaria control research project in Sri Lanka from 1980 to 1986. World Health Organization, Geneva, Switzerland. SER Project Reports 4.

Simmons, R.; Elias, C. 1994. The study of client-provider interactions: a review of methodological issues. Studies in Family Planning, 25(1), 1–17.

Singer, M. 1994. AIDS and the health crisis of the U.S. urban poor: the perspective of critical medical anthropology. Social Science and Medicine, 39(7), 931–948.

Sivard, R.L. 1985. Women: a world survey. World Priorities, Washington, DC, USA. 44 pp.

Smart, C.; Smart, B. 1978. Women, sexuality and social control. Routledge and Kegan Paul, London, UK. 121 pp.

Soin, K. 1995. Gender, health, and sustainable development. In Hatcher Roberts, J.; Kitts, J.; Jones Arsenault, L., ed., Gender, health, and sustainable development: perspectives from Asia and the Caribbean. Proceedings of workshops held in Singapore, 23–26 January 1995, and in Bridgetown, Barbados, 6–9 December 1994. International Development Research Centre, Ottawa, ON, Canada. pp. 9–12.

Sotomayer, O.; Davalos, J.J.; Pena, C.F.; Urgel, R.; Melvy, A.; Vargas, B.; Pinto, O. 1994. Socioeconomic, cultural, and psychosocial factors of congenital Chagas' disease. In Wijeyaratne, P.; Hatcher Roberts, J.; Kitts, J.; Jones Arsenault, L., ed., Gender, health, and sustainable development: a Latin American perspective. Proceedings of a workshop held in Montevideo, Uruguay, 26–29 April 1994. International Development Research Centre, Ottawa, ON, Canada. pp. 115–124.

Stackhouse, J. 1995a. How the meek are earning their inheritance. Globe and Mail (Toronto), 4 February 1995, pp. D1–D2.

————— 1995b. A healthy interest in reading. Globe and Mail (Toronto), 24 July 1995, p. A7.

Stamp, P. 1989. Technology, gender, and power in Africa. International Development Research Centre, Ottawa, ON, Canada. IDRC-TS63e. 185 pp.

Standing, H.; Kisekka, M. 1989. Sexual behaviour in sub-Saharan Africa: a review and annotated bibliography. Overseas Development Administration, London, UK. 250 pp.

Status of Women Canada. 1994. Canada's national report to the United Nations for the Fourth World Conference on Women. Status of Women Canada, Ottawa, ON, Canada. 85 pp.

Stephenson, D. 1987. Davey and Lightbody's The control of disease in the tropics: a handbook for physicians and other workers in tropical and international community health (5th ed.). H.K. Lewis and Co. Ltd, London, UK. 509 pp.

Strebel, A. 1992. There's absolutely nothing I can do, just believe in God: South African women with AIDS. Agenda, 12, 50–62.

———— 1993. Women and AIDS: a study of issues in the prevention of HIV infection. Department of Psychology, University of Cape Town, South Africa. PhD thesis, 244 pp.

———— 1994. "It's difficult to leave your man over a condom": social understanding of AIDS and gender. In Wijeyaratne, P.; Jones Arsenault, L.; Hatcher Roberts, J.; Kitts, J., ed., Gender, health, and sustainable development: proceedings of a workshop held in Nairobi, Kenya, 5–8 October 1993. International Development Research Centre, Ottawa, ON, Canada. pp. 34–45.

Tan, L. 1995. Population development and reproductive health from a gender perspective. In Hatcher Roberts, J.; Kitts, J.; Jones Arsenault, L., ed., Gender, health, and sustainable development: perspectives from Asia and the Caribbean. Proceedings of workshops held in Singapore, 23–26 January 1995, and in Bridgetown, Barbados, 6–9 December 1994. International Development Research Centre, Ottawa, ON, Canada. pp. 139–142.

Tandon, V. 1995. Macroparasitic infections in Meghalaya, North-East India. In Hatcher Roberts, J.; Kitts, J.; Jones Arsenault, L., ed., Gender, health, and sustainable development: perspectives from Asia and the Caribbean. Proceedings of workshops held in Singapore, 23–26 January 1995, and in Bridgetown, Barbados, 6–9 December 1994. International Development Research Centre, Ottawa, ON, Canada. pp. 143–150.

Tekle-Haimanot, R.; Forsgren, L.; Gebrre-Mariam, A.; Abebe, M.; Holgrem, G.; Heibel, J.; Ekstedt, J. 1992. Attitudes of rural people in central Ethiopia towards leprosy and a brief comparison with observations on epilepsy. Leprosy Review, 63, 157.

Thakur, C.P. 1981. Kala-azar hits again. Journal of Tropical Medicine and Hygiene, 84(66).

Thompson, E. 1995. Opening address. In Hatcher Roberts, J.; Kitts, J.; Jones Arsenault, L., ed., Gender, health, and sustainable development: perspectives from Asia and the Caribbean. Proceedings of workshops held in Singapore, 23–26 January 1995, and in Bridgetown, Barbados, 6–9 December 1994.

International Development Research Centre, Ottawa, ON, Canada. pp. 251–255.

Thomson, C. 1994. Play it safe, and don't panic. The Bulletin (Brussels), 24 November 1994, p. 26.

Thurman, O.; Franklin, K. 1990. AIDS and college health: knowledge, threat, and prevention from a northeastern university. Journal of American College Health, 38, 179–184.

Tillett, T. 1994. Opening address — Health policy research in Latin America and the Caribbean: the role of the household. In Wijeyaratne, P.; Hatcher Roberts, J.; Kitts, J.; Jones Arsenault, L., ed., Gender, health, and sustainable development: a Latin American perspective. Proceedings of a workshop held in Montevideo, Uruguay, 26–29 April 1994. International Development Research Centre, Ottawa, ON, Canada. pp. 7–16.

Timoteo, C.C.; Llanos-Cuentas, A. 1994. Gender differentials in the acquisition of forest leishmaniasis. In Wijeyaratne, P.; Hatcher Roberts, J.; Kitts, J.; Jones Arsenault, L., ed., Gender, health, and sustainable development: a Latin American perspective. Proceedings of a workshop held in Montevideo, Uruguay, 26–29 April 1994. International Development Research Centre, Ottawa, ON, Canada. pp. 125–133.

Timyan, J.; Griffey Brechin, S.J.; Measham, D.M.; Ogunleye, B. 1993. Access to care: more than a problem of distance. In Koblinsky, M.; Timyan, J.; Gay, J., ed., The health of women: a global perspective. Westview Press, Boulder, CO, USA. pp. 217–234.

Tin Tin Saw, D. 1995. Availabilty of health providers to female clients. In Hatcher Roberts, J.; Vlassoff, C., ed., The female client and the health-care provider. International Development Research Centre, Ottawa, ON, Canada. p. 156.

Tomasevski, K. 1993. Women and human rights. Zed Books Ltd, London, UK. 162 pp.

Tsikata, D. 1994. Environmental degradation, gender and health in Ghana. In Wijeyaratne, P.; Jones Arsenault, L.; Hatcher Roberts, J.; Kitts, J., ed., Gender, health, and sustainable development: proceedings of a workshop held in Nairobi, Kenya, 5–8 October 1993. International Development Research Centre, Ottawa, ON, Canada. pp. 150–162.

Turmen, T.; AbouZahr, C. 1994. Safe motherhood. International Journal of Gynaecology and Obstetrics, 46, 143–153.

Udipi, S.A.; Varghese, M.A. 1995. Improving women's quality of life: enhancing self-image and increasing decision-making power. In Hatcher Roberts, J.; Kitts, J.; Jones Arsenault, L., ed., Gender, health, and sustainable development: perspectives from Asia and the Caribbean. Proceedings of workshops held in Singapore, 23–26 January 1995, and in Bridgetown, Barbados, 6–9 December 1994. International Development Research Centre, Ottawa, ON, Canada. pp. 151–160.

Ulin, P. 1992. African women and AIDS: negotiating behavioural change. Social Science and Medicine, 34(1), 63–73.

Ulrich, M.; Zulueta, A.; Caceres-Dittmar, G.; Sampson, C.; Pinardi, M.; Rada, E.M.; Aranzazu, N. 1992. Leprosy in women: characteristics and repercussions. In Wijeyaratne, P.; Rathgeber, E.M.; St.-Onge, E., ed., Women and tropical diseases. International Development Research Centre, Ottawa, ON, Canada. pp. 5–23.

UN (United Nations). 1991. Women: challenges to the year 2000. UN, New York, NY, USA. 96 pp.

————— 1994. Report of the International Conference on Population and Development, 5–13 September 1994, Cairo, Egypt. UN, New York, NY, USA. A/CONF.171/13, 115 pp.

————— 1995. The world's women 1995: trends and statistics. UN, New York, NY, USA. 188 pp.

UNDIESA (United Nations Department of International Economic and Social Affairs). 1991. The world's women: trends and statistics 1970–1990. UNDIESA, UN, New York, NY, USA. 120 pp.

UNDP (United Nations Development Programme). 1992. Young women: silence, susceptibility and HIV infection. Age and gender as independent variables in the acquisition of HIV. UNDP, New York, NY, USA. 8 pp.

UNFPA (United Nations Fund for Population Activities). 1990. The state of the world population. UNFPA, New York, NY, USA. 15 pp.

UNICEF (United Nations Children's Fund). 1987. The invisible adjustment: poor women and the economic crisis. Alfabeta, Santiago, Chile. 262 pp.

Usher, A.D. 1992. After the forest: AIDS as ecological collapse in Thailand. Development Dialogue, 1/2, 13–49.

van der Kwaak, A. 1992. Female circumcision and gender identity: a questionable alliance? Social Science and Medicine, 35, 777–787.

Vézina, N.; Tierney, D.; Messing, K. 1992. When is light work heavy? Components of the physical workload of sewing machine operators which may lead to health problems. Applied Ergonomics, 23, 268–276.

Vickers, J. 1991. Women and the world economic crisis. Zed Books Ltd, London, UK. 146 pp.

Vlassoff, C. 1994. Gender inequalities in health in the Third World: unchartered ground. Social Science and Medicine, 39(9) 1249–1259.

Vlassoff, C.; Bonilla, E. 1994. Gender-related differences in the impact of tropical diseases on women: what do we know? Journal of Biosocial Science, 26, 37–53.

Waring, M. 1993. The exclusion of women from "work" and opportunity. In Mahoney, K.E.; Mahoney, P., ed., Human rights in the twenty-first century. Kluwer Academic Publishers, The Hague, Netherlands. pp. 109–117.

Warren, K.S.; Bundy, D.A.P.; Anderson, R.M.; Jamison, D.T.; Pescott, N.; Senft, A. 1993. Helminth infection. In Jamieson, D.T.; Mosley, W.H.; Measham, A.R.; Bobadilla, J.L., ed., Disease control priorities in developing countries. Oxford Medical Publications, London, UK. pp. 131–160.

WASH Field Report. 1988. Nigeria maternal morbidity from guinea worm and child survival. Bureau for Science and Technology, United States Agency for

International Development, Washington, DC, USA. WASH Activity 424, 1–42.

Waterfield, R.L. 1981. The effect of posture on the volume of the leg. Journal of Physiology, 72, 131–136.

Watts, S.J.; Brieger, W.R.; Yacoob, M. 1989. Guinea worm: an in-depth study of what happens to mothers, families and communities. Social Science and Medicine, 29, 1043–1049.

Wawer, M.J. 1991. Dynamics of spread of HIV-1 infection in a rural district of Uganda. British Medical Journal, 303, 1303–1306.

WCED (World Commission on Environment and Development). 1987. Our common future. Oxford University Press, Oxford, UK. 383 pp.

Wee, V. 1995. Workshop objectives. In Hatcher Roberts, J.; Kitts, J.; Jones Arsenault, L., ed., Gender, health, and sustainable development: perspectives from Asia and the Caribbean. Proceedings of workshops held in Singapore, 23–26 January 1995, and in Bridgetown, Barbados, 6–9 December 1994. International Development Research Centre, Ottawa, ON, Canada. pp. 6–8.

Weitz, R. 1982. Feminist consciousness raising, self-concept, and depression. Sex Roles, 8, 231–241.

Werrbach, J.; Gilbert, L.A. 1987. Men, gender stereotyping, and psychotherapy: therapists perceptions of male clients. Professional Psychology, 18, 562–566.

WHO (World Health Organization). 1984. Biomass fuel combustion and health. WHO, Geneva, Switzerland.

———— 1990. Control of the leishmaniasis: report of a WHO expert committee. WHO, Geneva, Switzerland. Technical Report Series 793. 131 pp.

———— 1991. Tropical diseases: progress in research 1989–1990. Tenth programme report: Tropical Disease Research (TDR). WHO, Geneva, Switzerland.

———— 1993. Malaria worsens world-wide. Third World Resurgence, 29/30, 15–16.

———— 1994a. AIDS: images of the epidemic. WHO, Geneva, Switzerland. 142 pp.

———— 1994b. Women's health: towards a better world. Global Commission on Women's Health, WHO, Geneva, Switzerland. 20 pp.

———— 1995. Quality of health care for women: report of a workshop held in Budapest, Hungary, 15–17 October 1994. WHO, Geneva, Switzerland.

WHO; UNDP (World Health Organization; United Nations Development Programme). 1994. Women and AIDS: agenda for action. WHO, Geneva, Switzerland. 11 pp.

Wijeyaratne, P.; Jones Arsenault, L.K.; Murphy, C.J. 1994. Endemic disease and development: the leishmaniasis. Acta Tropica, 56, 349–364.

Wilson, J. 1993. Women as carers. In Berer, M.; Ray, S., ed., Women and HIV/AIDS: an international resource book. Pandora, London, UK. pp. 287–288.

Winch, P.J.; Lloyd, L.S.; Hoemeke, L.; Leontsini, E. 1994. Vector control at the household level: an analysis of its impact on women. Acta Tropica, 56, 327–329.

Win May, D.; Tun Sein, T.; Thet Wai, K.; Ni Aye, N. 1995. Traditional customs, cultural beliefs, and perceptions toward antenatal care in rural Myanmar: a qualitative approach. In Hatcher Roberts, J.; Kitts, J.; Jones Arsenault, L., ed.,

Gender, health, and sustainable development: perspectives from Asia and the Caribbean. Proceedings of workshops held in Singapore, 23–26 January 1995, and in Bridgetown, Barbados, 6–9 December 1994. International Development Research Centre, Ottawa, ON, Canada. pp. 180–190.

World Bank. 1993. World development report 1993: investing in health. Oxford University Press, London, UK. 329 pp.

————— 1995. World development report 1995: workers in an integrated world. Oxford University Press, London, UK. 254 pp.

Wyatt, H.V. 1995. The female client and the health provider: using poliomyelitis as a marker. In Hatcher Roberts, J.; Vlassoff, C., ed., The female client and the health-care provider. International Development Research Centre, Ottawa, ON, Canada. p. 159.

Wyss, K.; Nandjingar, M. 1995. Problems of utilization of nutritional rehabilitation services by mothers of malnourished children in N'Djamena (Chad). In Hatcher Roberts, J.; Vlassoff, C., ed., The female client and the health-care provider. International Development Research Centre, Ottawa, ON, Canada. pp. 138–153.

Yack, D. 1992. The use and value of qualitative methods in health research in developing countries. Social Science and Medicine, 35(4), 603–612.

Yen, N.Y. 1995. Gender, health, and sustainable development. In Hatcher Roberts, J.; Kitts, J.; Jones Arsenault, L., ed., Gender, health, and sustainable development: perspectives from Asia and the Caribbean. Proceedings of workshops held in Singapore, 23–26 January 1995, and in Bridgetown, Barbados, 6–9 December 1994. International Development Research Centre, Ottawa, ON, Canada. pp. 85–89.

Yudomustopo, H. 1995. Women and their perceptions of environment and health. In Hatcher Roberts, J.; Kitts, J.; Jones Arsenault, L., ed., Gender, health, and sustainable development: perspectives from Asia and the Caribbean. Proceedings of workshops held in Singapore, 23–26 January 1995, and in Bridgetown, Barbados, 6–9 December 1994. International Development Research Centre, Ottawa, ON, Canada. pp. 191–205.

Zajac, A. 1992. Clinicopathologic and socioeconomic impact of Chagas' disease on women: a review. In Wijeyaratne, P.; Rathgeber, E.M.; St.-Onge, E., ed., Women and tropical diseases. International Development Research Centre, Ottawa, ON, Canada. pp. 134–148.

Zhang, K. 1994. Health care for women in developing countries must be culturally sensitive. Paper presented at the workshop on the quality of health care for women in developing countries, 15–17 October 1994, Budapest, Hungary. World Health Organization, Geneva, Switzerland. 10 pp.

The Authors

Jennifer Kitts is a lawyer, with expertise in the health, legal, ethical, and socioeconomic issues affecting the lives of women. She worked as a research analyst and project manager with the Canadian Royal Commission on New Reproductive Technologies and has worked as a researcher, writer, and editor, specializing in women's health issues, with IDRC, the World Health Organization, and the Community Health Research Unit of the University of Ottawa in Ottawa, Canada. She is currently completing a Master of Laws (LLM) in international and comparative law at the University of Brussels in Belgium and will be returning to Canada in September 1996 to work with the Ethics and Legal Affairs Division of the Canadian Medical Association.

Janet Hatcher Roberts is a health-policy specialist in the Program Branch of IDRC. Her training and expertise is in anthropology, nursing, epidemiology, and health policy. She has worked as an assistant professor in community health and epidemiology, as a policy analyst with the federal government and at the provincial and district levels, and, before joining IDRC, as the Deputy Director of Research and Evaluation at the Canadian Royal Commission on New Reproductive Technologies. She has been a long-time advocate in the area of women's health, running two local offices and sitting on the national board of DES ACTION.

About the Institution

The International Development Research Centre (IDRC) is committed to building a sustainable and equitable world. IDRC funds developing-world researchers, thus enabling the people of the South to find their own solutions to their own problems. IDRC also maintains information networks and forges linkages that allow Canadians and their developing-world partners to benefit equally from a global sharing of knowledge. Through its actions, IDRC is helping others to help themselves.

About the Publisher

IDRC Books publishes research results and scholarly studies on global and regional issues related to sustainable and equitable development. As a specialist in development literature, IDRC Books contributes to the body of knowledge on these issues to further the cause of global understanding and equity. IDRC publications are sold through its head office in Ottawa, Canada, as well as by IDRC's agents and distributors around the world.